HYPOTHYROIDISM,

HEALTH

&

HAPPINESS

HYPOTHYROIDISM,
HEALTH
&
HAPPINESS

The RIDDLE *of*
ILLNESS
REVEALED

STEVEN F. HOTZE, MD

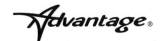

Published by Advantage, Charleston, South Carolina.
Member of Advantage Media Group.

ADVANTAGE is a registered trademark and the Advantage colophon is a trademark of Advantage Media Group, Inc.

Printed in the United States of America.

ISBN: 978-159932-396-1
LCCN: 2013936084

This publication is designed to provide accurate and authoritative information in regard to the subject matter covered. It is sold with the understanding that the publisher is not engaged in rendering legal, accounting, or other professional services. If legal advice or other expert assistance is required, the services of a competent professional person should be sought.

Notice: This book is intended as a reference guide, not as a medical manual. The information given here is designed to help you make informed decisions about your health. It is not intended as a substitute for any treatment that may have been prescribed to your by your doctor or therapist. If you suspect that you have a medical or emotional problem, we urge you to seek competent medical or psychiatric help.

The names of some of those whose cases are presented in this book have been changed to preserve their privacy.

Advantage Media Group is proud to be a part of the Tree Neutral® program. Tree Neutral offsets the number of trees consumed in the production and printing of this book by taking proactive steps such as planting trees in direct proportion to the number of trees used to print books. To learn more about Tree Neutral, please visit **www.treeneutral.com**. To learn more about Advantage's commitment to being a responsible steward of the environment, please visit **www.advantagefamily.com/green**

Advantage Media Group is a publisher of business, self-improvement, and professional development books and online learning. We help entrepreneurs, business leaders, and professionals share their Stories, Passion, and Knowledge to help others Learn & Grow™. Do you have a manuscript or book idea that you would like us to consider for publishing? Please visit **advantagefamily.com** or call **1.866.775.1696**.

This book is dedicated to Richard Mabray, MD, mentor and friend, who introduced me to Broda Barnes', MD, method of evaluating and treating hypothyroid individuals.

ACKNOWLEDGMENTS

When I first wrote *Hormones, Health, and Happiness*, I felt very strongly that it carried an important message of hope. Since it was published in 2005, we have been able to serve tens of thousands of patients, or "guests," at the Hotze Health & Wellness Center, helping them regain their health and get their lives back. *Hormones, Health, and Happiness* was written for all those who, like you, were sick and tired of being sick and tired and were willing to make changes in their lives.

This second book, *Hypothyroidism, Health, and Happiness,* has also been written for you. We all have the seeds of greatness within us and the desire to discover our unique ability so that we can better ourselves and create value for others. If we are in a state of poor health, we cannot reach our goals. It is my hope that you will find the information within these pages both educational and encouraging, and that it will help you, as well as your family, friends, and associates onto the pathway of success.

Anyone who knows what is entailed in writing a book realizes that there are numerous people behind the scenes who are also responsible for bringing this book to fruition, so I would like to take the opportunity to thank them.

My mother, Margaret Hotze, is one of the strongest women I know. She has been a constant source of inspiration to me throughout my life. She raised me in a Christian home and made sure that my faith in Jesus Christ was cultivated by providing me with a Catholic education from the first through the twelfth grade. Mom graduated from the University of Texas with a journalism degree and has been a lifelong, prolific writer. Of course, she is the one who taught me to write. She also instructed me to think independently and not follow the herd. I admire her and love her dearly.

The influence that my father, Ernest Hotze, had on me continues to impact my life. Dad never knew a stranger. He was an enthusiastic salesman and entrepreneur. Dad founded Compressor Engineering Corporation (CECO) in 1964, and it is still being managed by four of my brothers. CECO employs more than 400 people. Dad left his eight children and 46 grandchildren a rich heritage.

Janie is my beautiful, loving, dedicated wife of 44 years, mother of our eight children and 17 grandchildren. She has not only joyfully raised our large family, but she also worked at the Hotze Health & Wellness Center in the early, critical years of our growth. Her consistency, dedication, and belief in me have provided me with the encouragement that I have needed to pursue my goals. She is my number-one cheerleader.

Monica Luedecke, president of Hotze Enterprises, has worked with me for the past 22-plus years and has made herself an indispensable leader of our organization. She set the goal for writing this book and played a key role in its composition. She has driven this book project from start to finish, writing, editing, developing an inside and outside team to work on the book, contracting with the publisher, and making sure we met our deadlines. If it weren't for Monica, this book would not be available to you or to the millions of people who will benefit from understanding how hypothyroidism adversely affects every area of your body. Knowing this may enable you to solve the riddle of your illness. Because of Monica's disciplined, diligent efforts, this book has come to life and will guide millions of people to restoring their health, transforming their lives, and improving their worlds, naturally.

When this book was in its first stage, a talented young lady, Jenny Perot, worked on the initial draft. I am grateful for her diligent efforts.

Stacey Bandfield, my director of scheduling, was instrumental in the completion of this book. Stacey assisted with the review and editing of each chapter and most importantly, helped me to budget the time necessary to complete this project. Meanwhile, her assistant, Pam Whitfield, played a key role in identifying and referencing the numerous sources in this book. I am most grateful for their help.

The excellent team at Advantage Media, especially Adam Witty, its founder and CEO, Sonya Giffin, and Alison Morse professionally guided us through the steps to publishing this book. Denis Boyles, Brooke White, and Rich Laliberte evaluated and performed the final edit of this book, putting the polish on it so that it would shine.

Gina Teafatiller, our chief marketing officer, worked with Advantage Media to create a timeline for publication of this book, developed the book cover design and managed the entire marketing process. This was no small feat and required a yeoman's effort to make this happen. I am very grateful to her for her tireless efforts.

I would also like to thank Richard Mabray, MD, Julian Whitaker, MD, Thierry Hertoghe, MD, Erika Schwartz, MD, and David Brownstein, MD, all of whom have encouraged and inspired me on my pathway of providing natural approaches to health.

My colleagues Dr. David Sheridan and Dr. Donald Ellsworth are brilliant and passionate about serving our guests at the Hotze Health & Wellness Center, as are our nurse practitioner Debbie Janak, and physician assistant Amber Littler. They and our entire team of health care professionals have a heart for service. They have partnered with our guests to help them onto the pathway of health and wellness so that they can obtain and maintain health and wellness naturally and get their lives back. Without this great team of professionals, we would be unable to provide the expertise and hospitality that give our guests hope.

All of the people whom I have mentioned so far are owed a deep debt of gratitude for their inspiration and their efforts. It is the guests, however, who were willing to share their personal stories of restored health who really made *Hypothyroidism, Health, and Happiness* possible. They took time out of their busy schedules to be interviewed so that their experiences could help others. Though we were unable to include all of the stories told by our guests in this book, I extend my heartfelt thanks to all the guests who were interviewed or who submitted their story to us.

The guests at the Hotze Health & Wellness Center have chosen to take charge of their lives and make an investment in their health. They keep me and all the 90-plus members of my staff focused on our vision of leading a "wellness revolution" that will change the way women and men are treated in midlife through the use of natural, bioidentical hormones, and natural approaches to health. Our guests are a constant reminder that good health is essential to experiencing an enjoyable and fulfilling life. We have a moral duty to partner with as many people as possible in order to help them enjoy a better quality of life.

We have been contacted by over 100,000 individuals who have told us their stories of faltering health and how it has drained the enjoyment from their lives. While each person has a unique personal story, the symptoms they express are very similar. There is a common thread running throughout the stories of most of these individuals and that is the thread of undiagnosed hypothyroidism.

This book was written for you. Please take it to heart. It may change your life.

TABLE OF CONTENTS

LOST WISDOM

Modern medicine with its advanced technologies and pharmaceuticals seems a far cry from medicine during the late nineteenth century—and it is. But that doesn't mean the practices of medical pioneers have no relevance for us today. In fact, the startling truth is that certain early insights continue to have a direct but unappreciated bearing on many health conditions that plague people in the twenty-first century. What's more, tracing our understanding of how specific discoveries and practices came to evolve can offer valuable lessons that have been overlooked and all but lost in the fog of time.

Medical science was in its infancy back in the late 1800s but was rapidly advancing. Nowhere was this truer than in England, where a prominent group of physicians had established an organization called the Clinical Society of London. Society physicians would meet on a periodic basis to discuss medical issues of the time. In the early 1880s the society set about investigating a medical mystery that sprang from an intriguing set of clinical observations that all converged at once.

At that time, a number of individuals—most of them women— were being brought to the society with symptoms and signs that appeared related to similar symptoms and signs that the physicians saw in cretinoid individuals, or cretins.

The term *cretin* today has connotations of stupidity or loutish behavior. But in those days, cretinism didn't relate so much to character as to an observable set of clinical traits. *Cretin* was a term applied to individuals who did not develop properly from childhood. They weren't midgets or dwarfs, but were physically small in stature and had certain characteristic features such as an enlarged tongue, oversized head, and puffy skin. In addition, cretins never developed mentally or emotionally.

In some cases, young cretins had a goiter—an enlargement of a gland in their neck that we now know as the thyroid gland. The thyroid gland produces hormones that are vital in maintaining normal growth and governing the body's metabolism. In nineteenth-century Europe, however, doctors had no idea what the gland did. They theorized that fluid in the gland was important for the functioning of the body, that it stimulated the nervous system, or that it reduced toxins in the body. But the existence of hormones and the idea that deficiency of an organ-derived substance could make you sick was foreign to the medical profession of the day.

Yet physicians were piecing together elements of a puzzle that would eventually lead to significant advances in the understanding and treatment of hormone-related conditions. Doctors knew that cretinism was somehow related to the thyroid gland. And now, with the cases coming to the society, they knew that adult women who had already developed physically, mentally, and emotionally could, in midlife, develop physical signs that made them similar in many ways to cretinoid individuals.

What was this malady in adults? What caused it? What did cretins and previously healthy women with similar symptoms share in common? The society formed a committee to do a five-year study probing these questions. Headed by a physician named William

Ord, the committee sent letters to prominent physicians throughout the United Kingdom, asking if they'd seen patients with the distinguishing cretinoid symptoms. Plenty of them had. Eventually, the society's committee evaluated 109 cases described by different medical professionals.

WORD WISE

Clinical: Though often used interchangeably to mean "medical," the term *clinical* refers to a specific form of medical care that's based on actual treatment and observation of patients in the clinic or at the bedside. This hands-on approach makes clinical care more personal and experienced-based than theoretical or experimental medicine, though all of these aspects of care tend to be interdependent.

AN UNKNOWN ENTITY

When the committee finally delivered its report to a regular meeting of the Clinical Society of London in May 1888, the session was unusually packed. Some attendees came from as far away as the United States. The report not only drew on clinical observations from Britain, but reports from throughout Europe. Its title referenced the "Subject of Myxedema," a term that Ord coined to describe swelling due to a thick mucus-like substance that pathologic examination found under the skin of patients who had not survived their afflictions. Myxedema was a wholly new clinical entity that had not been previously described. And while Ord's term is not widely known outside medical circles, the condition his group reported and defined still reverberates a century and a quarter later. Some of the observations that highlighted the condition were these:

- It afflicted six times more women than men.
- In every case in which a pathological exam was done after death, the patient's thyroid gland was found to be abnormal—often scarred, damaged, degenerated, or destroyed. In many cases, the gland was completely nonfunctioning.
- Patients experienced a wide range of symptoms, including major signs of cretinism such as enlarged tongue, puffy or pale skin, and brittle fingernails. But patients also experienced more subtle symptoms that continue to resonate with many women in the twenty-first century. These include fatigue, difficulty with weight, sensitivity to the cold (especially in the hands and feet), inability to focus or think clearly (what many patients now describe as "brain fog"), insomnia, poor sleep habits, mood swings, depression, panic attacks, anxiety, constipation, irritable bowel function, hair loss, recurring chronic infections, and disturbed menstrual cycles.

Beyond the clinical description, committee physicians reported a number of significant observations from across the Western world that further illuminated the role of the thyroid gland and ultimately shed light on treatment.

For example, animal studies found that when the thyroid gland was surgically removed (a procedure known as a thyroidectomy), animals would develop symptoms such as low body temperature and slow metabolism, gradually—but prematurely—deteriorating and dying. It was the same story in people. When physicians treated goiters by taking out the thyroid gland, patients deteriorated, developing signs and symptoms of myxedema and typically dying within a year or two. While tragic for these unfortunate patients, this finding provided another advance in understanding and made clear that people could not survive without thyroid function. In countries such as Switzerland, Germany, and Austria, where goiters were particularly common, a physician who noted the quick decline of thyroidectomy patients tried a different approach: removing only a portion of the thyroid. Those patients did better.

THE ADVENT OF THYROID REPLACEMENT

Still, the society's committee report had no clear answers on treatment. Thyroidectomy results seemed mixed. Giving stimulants to rev the metabolism didn't help much either. But the five-year work of Ord's group provided the groundwork for another important development three years later. Realizing the importance of thyroid function, a physician named George Redmayne Murray treated a 46-year-old woman with myxedema by injecting her with an extract of sheep thyroid. He called his treatment "organotherapy." A variation of the technique had been practiced centuries earlier in ancient China, but colleagues scoffed at Murray's approach even though the patient improved dramatically. (In fact, she went on to live a full life, dying at age 74 in 1921.) After Murray published his results, others started reporting similar successes with thyroid replacement.

Thyroid treatments improved even more in the years leading up to and beyond the turn of the century. Because injectable sheep extract was difficult to prepare, physicians instead began using dried, or desiccated, thyroid, which was effective, stable, easier to work with, and relatively inexpensive. Clinicians refined dosages so that patients wouldn't receive too much too soon, and an apothecary system of measures was developed to guide prescriptions. Diagnosis and treatment were based on clinical observation: If patients exhibited symptoms typical of thyroid-related problems, doctors would begin thyroid replacement. If patients got well, that verified the diagnosis.

As Europe descended into World War I, thyroid research produced more breakthroughs. Thyroid hormone—or what was later found to be one major form of it, called thyroxin—was discovered, and its chemical structure was described. The severe extremes of myxedema and a spectrum of symptoms leading up to it came to be understood as low-thyroid disorders—what today is known as hypothyroidism.

Throughout the first half of the twentieth century, natural desiccated thyroid was the front-line treatment of hypothyroidism, which was diagnosed and treated based on clinical observation. Desiccated thyroid was "natural" in the sense that it came from actual thyroid glands, typically from pigs. In fact, the well-known meatpacking company, Armour, was a major supplier. Not every doctor was attuned to the problem of hypothyroidism, but those who were often saw the health of patients who received thyroid improve dramatically.

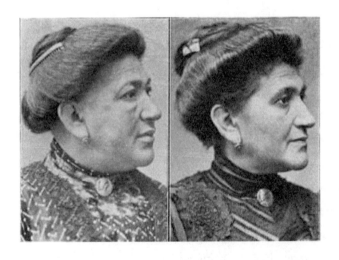

Source: Hertoghe, E. Medical Record, Sep. 1914, Vol.86, Issue 12, 489-505.

If patients exhibited symptoms typical of thyroid-related problems, doctors would begin thyroid replacement. If patients got well, that verified the diagnosis.

A FUNDAMENTAL CHANGE IN APPROACH

Today many physicians still aren't aware of the profound role that thyroid hormones play in health. This book will show you just how important proper thyroid care can be for a wide range of maladies that remain widespread despite the foundations of thyroid treatment that were laid more than a century ago. It will also show the way that deeply ingrained elements of modern medicine may actually be making many patients' problems worse.

As we'll see, a fundamental shift in thyroid care has taken place that has distanced it from the promising beginnings that led to decades of effective thyroid treatment through the middle of the last century. Starting in the 1960s, drug companies came out with synthetic thyroid preparations and heavily promoted them. Natural desiccated thyroid gradually became less popular among physicians, and synthetic thyroid has become the drug of choice among endocrinologists and other doctors who treat thyroid conditions.

We'll examine why growing numbers of doctors—and especially patients—are beginning to demand more natural treatments that are truer to the roots of thyroid care established by Ord, Murray, and other pioneers. We'll see how hypothyroidism is responsible for many prevalent conditions, yet still is often overlooked. And we'll examine how a medical culture that discourages independent thinking reinforces a model of care that fails to help a great number of people who might otherwise lead better, healthier, more productive lives.

INTRODUCTION
LOW THYROID NATION

My people perish from a lack of knowledge.

—HOSEA 4:6

The premise of this book is that the decline in the health of the American public, and more specifically, the decline in your health, is primarily caused by hypothyroidism.

That assertion is based on clinical observation, research, and problems associated with current practices in medical profession. This book offers both a challenge and a prescription. And a challenge of today's medicine begins with a fundamental question: Has medicine's current view of how health problems should be diagnosed and treated made Americans healthier, happier, and more productive? Let's take a brief overview of America's health status, and then you decide:

- If the system of medical care in our country were working, why are 67 percent of Americans overweight and 33 percent obese? Compare this to an obesity rate of 8 percent in Italy and nine percent in France where pasta and bread are served at every meal. This means that obesity is four times more prevalent in the United States than in Italy and France. In fact, the United States has the highest incidence of obesity of any country in the world.

- This problem with overweight and obesity has led to dramatic increases in the incidence of type 2 diabetes (formerly known as adult onset diabetes), high blood pressure, heart disease, degenerative arthritis, Alzheimer's disease, and cancer.

- Health care costs have increased ten times since 1980, from $256 billion to $2.6 trillion in 2010,[1] and health care spending now encompasses nearly one-fifth of the gross national product.[2]

This has led to dramatic increases in insurance premiums, which threaten the financial stability of both individuals and businesses. The cost of business-sponsored health care plans has doubled since 2002.[3] Meanwhile, Medicare and Medicaid expenditures have increased dramatically as well, threatening the financial solvency of state and federal governments.

We are an unhealthy people, an unhealthy nation. Our population is becoming sicker and sicker. We are spending more and more on the same failed disease model of medicine and getting the same results or worse. It will inevitably lead to our bankruptcy and our downfall as a nation unless we make a dramatic change in our course of action.

What has caused this terrible decline in health that we are experiencing in America? Why do we have an epidemic of obesity, diabetes, high blood pressure, heart disease, degenerative arthritis, gastrointestinal problems, and cancer? Is there a common thread among these health problems that would lead us to the underlying cause of these varied health problems and the diversity of symptoms with which they are associated?

I believe there are indeed a number of common threads—and I'll detail them in the pages that follow. Throughout this book, you'll repeatedly encounter several themes and find them reinforced in a variety of different ways. If you take these themes to heart and adopt the principles that I advocate for obtaining and maintaining health naturally, you will have the opportunity to restore your health and transform your life. When this happens, you will want to join forces with me to bring about a wellness revolution in America.

It all gets down to personal responsibility. Neither the state and federal governments nor the insurance companies, nor your employer, are responsible for your health. You and you alone are responsible. So, if you are willing to take personal responsibility for your health, this book is for you.

Revolutions always challenge the current establishment structure that controls the power in society. In our society today, that means challenging the way medicine is practiced under the strong influence of the pharmaceutical and insurance industries. It also means challenging the way doctors view some of our most common yet vexing health problems.

Here are some of the key themes that I'll be referencing and building upon:

> *We are spending more and more on the same failed disease model of medicine and getting the same results—or worse.*

1. America is a hypothyroid nation.

Wherever I go, I look at the sea of faces that carry the marks of hypothyroidism at airports, hotels, restaurants, barber shops, grocery stores, sporting events, and church services. These individuals are leading their lives totally unaware that the symptoms that plague them are a result of their low thyroid condition.

It's heartbreaking.

Living with hypothyroidism means that these individuals will never fully enjoy the life that God intended for them to experience. They will be tired, subject to recurrent and chronic infections and diseases, depressed, overweight, and prone to stress, and will ultimately become spectators in life rather than fully engaged participants.

Hypothyroidism does not discriminate. It affects people living at all socioeconomic levels, whether they are struggling financially or have achieved the highest pinnacle of success, whether they are a celebrities or one in a cast of thousands. It is a common condition, and yet it commonly goes undiagnosed or misdiagnosed. It is far easier for physicians to prescribe pharmaceutical drugs to treat the symptoms caused by hypothyroidism than it is for them to challenge current thinking and discover the underlying cause of the multiple symptoms experienced by those afflicted with unrecognized hypothyroidism.

WORD WISE

Hypothyroidism. The term *hypo* means abnormally decreased or deficient. *Hypothyroidism* refers to a condition marked by a lack of thyroid gland activity. Its most severe form is known as myxedema, the condition that William Ord and his colleagues first described in the 1880s, as outlined in the Prelude. Less severe forms of hypothyroidism, however, can cause a wide range of problems that are rampant in America today.

---

2. **Safe and effective treatments for hypothyroidism have been around for more than 100 years.**

We saw in the Prelude to this book how medical science long ago unraveled some of the fundamental mysteries about the important role that thyroid hormones play in good health and devised standards for effective treatment that were the standard of care for more than half a century. Yet mainstream medicine continues to ignore both the problems of hypothyroidism and many of its proven solutions.

The sad truth is that regardless of who you are or how much money you have, if you are not proactive and do not take charge of your health, you risk being misdiagnosed. This has happened to millions of individuals, and they and their families have suffered as a result.

This is so sad because it is so preventable. If you remember what it was like to be full of energy and vibrant with seemingly unlimited opportunities, but you now feel like a shadow of your former self, spiraling downward into poor health, you may benefit from long-established but underused thyroid treatments.

3. Americans are sick and tired of feeling sick and tired.

The symptoms of hypothyroidism are, in fact, so common that you may recognize them from your own personal experience. Tens of millions of others have as well—and as a nation, we are sick and tired of being sick and tired. Are you experiencing fatigue, unhealthy weight, insomnia, depressed moods, panic attacks, anxiety, brain fog, joint and muscle pain, constipation, gastrointestinal issues, tingling in your hands and feet, loss of libido, recurrent infections, menstrual irregularities, hair loss in females, dry skin or skin rashes, among others? If so, have you been told that your blood work is normal? Do you have a medicine cabinet full of drugs? If your answer to these questions is yes, what you are about to read in this book will resonate in your heart.

If we were to meet one year from now, what would have to change in your life for you to feel pleased about your health progress? Would it be fitting into a smaller dress or suit, securing a better job opportunity, having more quality time with your family and friends? Would you like to feel exceptional rather than just average? Would you rather experience more vitality, instead of feeling sick and tired of being sick and tired?

Within the pages of this book you will discover crucial information regarding the dramatic, adverse effects that hypothyroidism can have on the quality of your life. It is my hope that you will not only learn to identify its symptoms and seek treatment if you recognize yourself in these pages, but that you will learn to question conventional thinking and seek a different solution before you willingly accept every drug that is prescribed to you. If you are feeling unhealthy, it is not because you are deficient in pharmaceuticals. People are not sick and tired because they have low levels of drugs in their bodies.

4. **Physicians adhere to medical dogma.**

That's not surprising. Doctors are trained to be compliant and not question their academic professors. Anyone who challenges the current medical dogma is considered a heretic and ostracized by other physicians. Many physicians have forgotten or have never been trained to ask, "Why?" Even the most basic questions often go unasked:

- Why are some individuals prone to poor health and disease while others remain healthy and vital?
- Why do we use drugs to mask symptoms instead of getting at the root cause of the problem?
- Why is there such opposition in the medical field to natural approaches to health?

As a physician who has helped more than 25,000 patients to get their lives back, I am on a mission to lead a wellness revolution that will help millions of people who are completely unaware that they can obtain and maintain health and wellness naturally. The information in this book remains obscure to the masses, but now you have it in your hands. Tens of millions of people have also lost their health to poor habits and well-intentioned but misguided physicians who only offer pharmaceutical drugs to mask symptoms. You and only you can make the decision that will change your future by taking charge of your health.

Within these pages you will read inspirational stories about individuals like yourself who struggled with poor health but who chose get their health and their lives back. No matter what your state in life is—a student, a newlywed, a mom, a teacher, a politician, a business person, or a retiree—my goal for you is to give you the knowledge to help you restore your health, transform your life, and improve your world, naturally. Helping you understand the widespread epidemic of hypothyroidism and how it affects you and your family is a great place to start.

5. **The pharmaceutical and insurance industries dominate medicine.**

Treating symptoms is just what the pharmaceutical industry encourages doctors and patients to do. The willingness of physicians to prescribe drugs to patients in order to mask symptoms rather than diagnosing the underlying cause of those symptoms has created a nation of legal drug addicts who are slowly being poisoned to death by their medications. Just to name a few, antidepressants, antianxiety and sleep medication, addicting pain relievers, anti-cholesterol and anti-inflammatory drugs, amphetamines for so-called attention deficit disorders—all of which have severe side effects—are passed out like candy. This is a disaster of enormous proportions.

Support from the leadership of mainstream medicine has been purchased by these industries. Insurance companies control the doctors' patients and the doctors' incomes. Many medical societies and their leaders, as well as many academic medical professors, receive payment from the pharmaceutical and insurance companies to promote these industries to practicing physicians and to the public at large. Medical society journals are chock full of pharmaceutical advertisements. Medical society conferences are handsomely under-written by pharmaceutical companies.

The pharmaceutical companies have no interest in promoting natural approaches to health because this would undermine their business model of selling drugs to the public. And you can be sure that the pharmaceutical and insurance companies are calling the political shots in order to protect themselves from competition.

Likewise, insurance companies have no interest in promoting natural approaches to health. A healthy public would require less health care, causing insurance premiums to plummet. Health insurance companies are regulated by the 50 state boards of insurance that allow the companies to set their premium rates to insure that they make a fixed percent profit. With people becoming sicker from a rising incidence of high blood pressure, diabetes, heart disease, degenerative arthritis, gastrointestinal disorders, Alzheimer's disease, and cancer, the insurance premiums inevitably rise, increasing the revenues to the insurance companies. State insurance boards grant insurance companies the right to increase their premiums to ensure that they make a fixed percent profit. If you were the insurance company, would you rather make 15 percent profit on $5 billion in revenues from premiums, which would be $750 million, or 15 percent profit on $10 billion in revenues, which would be $1.5 billion?

Today you live in a culture where information is at your fingertips through the Internet, and yet you are probably unaware of the most basic ways that your body functions, and what to do about them. You may have relied too heavily on physicians who, although well intentioned, never get to the root cause of your symptoms, but instead manage them by prescribing drugs.

As you read this book, please keep in mind that information without action is worthless. Allow me to encourage you to find help for yourself and your loved ones today. Share this book widely with your family, associates, and friends. You will gain knowledge about your health that your doctor is probably unable to provide, not because he wants to keep you unhealthy, but because he has been trained since medical school that symptoms are to be managed through surgery or drugs.

MONEY TALKS

In 2011 pharmaceutical sales in the United States totaled $320 billion. With their huge profits, the pharmaceutical companies saturate the television airwaves with advertisements to seduce the uneducated public into using their drugs—and advertising pays off in spades. U.S. citizens, who make up only 5 percent of the world's population, consume more than 40 percent of the pharmaceutical drugs made in the world. With that kind of income, the pharmaceutical companies can hire thousands of paid lobbyists and give to campaigns in order to gain tremendous influence with the politicians of both parties. The old adage remains true: "He who pays the piper calls the tune."

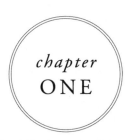

chapter
ONE

SETTING THE STAGE

PEGGY'S STORY

"Learn to live with it."

"**D**ear God, if my life is going to be like this, then I want a short life." This was the prayer that 51-year-old Peggy silently whispered.

The only future that she could envision was like a slippery downhill trail into a treacherous canyon shrouded with fog. Thoughts of happier years faded in her memory. Bone-throbbing exhaustion, unrelenting joint pain, "brain fog," weight gain, depressed moods, and insomnia had plagued her daily existence and had been worsening over the past several years. Now her symptoms seemed unbearable.

While driving to meet her next real estate client, Peggy reflected on what had caused her to have such a dismal outlook on the future. She wondered, "How has it come to this?" She had a terrific husband, a fine son, and successful real estate career, but her mind and body were falling apart at the seams. Peggy was just sick and tired of feeling sick and tired.

As a teenager, Peggy had been diagnosed with hypothyroidism, a low thyroid condition caused by a disorder called autoimmune thyroiditis. Peggy had taken Synthroid, a commonly prescribed synthetic thyroid drug, since that time. Unfortunately, Synthroid had provided her with little resolution of her hypothyroid symptoms.

Peggy's downhill slide began in earnest after she underwent a hysterectomy at the age of 38. Like many women, she was prescribed Premarin, a horse estrogen derived from pregnant mare's urine, after her surgery. That was when her symptoms of fatigue, depression, weight gain, difficulty thinking, and joint and muscle pain began to progressively worsen. It had occurred to Peggy that maybe she was not taking enough thyroid medication and that if her doctor would just give her a stronger dose, she might feel better. So she scheduled a doctor's appointment in order to discuss her health problems and have him check her thyroid hormone blood levels.

A MEDICAL NOT-SO-MERRY-GO-ROUND

Her doctor disinterestedly listened to her complaints and then said authoritatively, "Peggy, look, you have been on this same dose of thyroid for years and your blood tests have always been in the normal range. If you are taking your medication as I have instructed you to do, this time it will be no different. Your symptoms are not due to an inadequate thyroid dose."

During her follow-up office visit, Peggy's physician arrogantly informed her, "Your symptoms can't be due to your thyroid because your blood work is normal, just as I told you."

So, just as he had told thousands of his female patients before, he uttered his standard line, confidently asserting, "We find that most women like you benefit from an antidepressant." Then he just shook his head from side to side as if he were thinking, "These poor miserable women just can't keep it together."

Peggy countered, "But I am not depressed. I have a great marriage and a successful career. It's just that I don't feel well."

Standing erect in his starched white coat with a stethoscope dangling from his neck, her doctor sternly addressed her, "You may think that you are not depressed, but all your symptoms are classic for depression. That is why you need an antidepressant."

Shrugging his shoulders, her doctor told her in an unsympathetic tone, "You just need to learn to live with it like the other women in my practice."

Peggy felt abandoned and deserted. "Doesn't anyone understand?" she thought.

She was also stunned by his comments and his dismissive attitude and thought, "He must think that I am a hypochondriac."

Then Peggy began to doubt herself. "Maybe I am having mental problems. My doctor wouldn't give me a psychiatric drug if he didn't think that something was wrong with me mentally."

What followed can best be described as a medical merry-go-round—only there was nothing merry about it. With no other alternative solution known to her, Peggy began taking her antidepressant, but she found that she felt worse. She made another appointment to discuss this further downward spiral with her doctor. At the visit, her doctor smugly told her, "This proves that you need an antidepressant. We just need to make some adjustments in the dose." After increasing her dose, he sent her on her way.

There was no improvement. There were more doctor visits. There were different antidepressants and combinations of antidepressants prescribed.

INTO THE DRUG FOG

None of the drugs resolved Peggy's symptoms, and worse, they created a whole new set of symptoms for which there were more drugs. There were always more drugs. Her depression worsened and was accompanied by extreme fatigue. The muscles and joints throughout her entire body ached. As a side effect of her pharmaceutical cocktails, Peggy developed high blood pressure and heart palpitations for which, of course, she was treated with more prescription drugs. She began to be plagued by recurrent sinus infections and was repeatedly prescribed multiple courses of antibiotics to treat them.

Peggy's health and life were deteriorating. It was as if she were seeing the world through a fog. Her sense of humor was gone. She began detaching herself from friends. After describing these symptoms to her physician, Peggy gained yet another diagnosis: attention deficit disorder (ADD). Adderall was added to the increasingly long list of drugs Peggy took on a daily basis. Adderall is an amphetamine. You might have heard it called an "upper." One of the side effects of Adderall is insomnia, which Peggy experienced, so a sleep medication was added to Peggy's list of drugs. Despite constant adjustments to every other prescription drug she was taking, her thyroid medication remained unchanged. Every physician who reviewed her thyroid lab work said, "Everything looks normal."

The irony was that Peggy couldn't even remember the last time she had felt normal.

She had seen the best doctors and numerous specialists: gynecologists, endocrinologists, internists, rheumatologists, psychiatrists, and so forth. None of them could tell her why she was having her symptoms. All they could offer her were more prescription drugs to mask them. She felt hopeless. She had lost faith in her physicians.

In spite of the serious and debilitating decline in her health, Peggy still managed her real estate business. She took naps between clients and scheduled all of her appointments in the morning to avoid the inevitable crash of afternoon fatigue. She did this because her physicians told her that this is what happened to women as they aged. They echoed her first doctor and told her that she would just have to learn to live with it.

A NEW BEGINNING

When Peggy visited the Hotze Health & Wellness Center, she told us that we were her last resort, and she was at the end of her rope. After listening to her describe her health issues, we validated her symptoms, affirmed her concerns, and told her we appreciated the opportunity to partner with her in her quest to restore her health. During an extended visit with one of our physicians, David Sheridan, MD, Peggy revealed that she was taking nine different drugs. This cascade of pharmaceuticals had started with synthetic thyroid medication. But despite taking it, Peggy continued to have symptoms of hypothyroidism.

This is the same story that we hear from every guest who has been put on synthetic thyroid drugs, namely, Synthroid, Levoxyl, or Levothroid. The reason is easily explained: these synthetic thyroid drugs do not contain the active thyroid hormone.[4]

Dr. Sheridan recommended that Peggy switch from the synthetic thyroid to a bioidentical thyroid hormone preparation: desiccated porcine thyroid. Desiccated thyroid is derived from pork thyroid and contains the identical thyroid hormones that your body makes: thyroxine (T4) and triiodothyronine (T3). Desiccated thyroid has been used for more than 100 years in medicine. It is safe, effective, and inexpensive.[5] Peggy's thyroid dose was adjusted based upon the resolution of her symptoms rather than her blood test.

Dr. Sheridan made a few additional recommendations for Peggy to replenish her depleted natural sex and adrenal hormones with the bioidentical hormones, progesterone, estrogen, and cortisol. Within a few months, Peggy had been weaned off her nine prescription drugs. The plethora of side effects caused by these drugs resolved, and Peggy began to feel terrific. After 13 years of being overmedicated with pharmaceutical drugs prescribed by mainstream medical doctors, Peggy finally had her life back.

MODERN MEDICINE CAN'T ANSWER WHY

Some 350 million people visit medical doctors each year. This is a large number, but here's an even more impressive figure: More than 420 million people visit alternative medicine practitioners each year. That is 70 million more visits from people who are choosing to look beyond current therapies to alternative medicine for answers to their health problems—and the trend is increasing daily.[6]

What has caused conventional medicine's fall from its pedestal? Enamored with a host of new drugs offered by the pharmaceutical industry and with innovations in medical technology, it seems that many physicians have forgotten the two most important rules in diagnosing a patient's problems:

1. Doctors should listen carefully to the patient's complaints and medical history, and evaluate their physical signs.
2. Doctors should ask themselves: "What is the underlying cause of these symptoms?"

It is much easier to prescribe a drug than it is to think. Thinking is hard and it takes time. That's partly why the patient's symptoms and physical signs have taken a back seat to blood tests.[7] Prior to the advent of technology, your doctor would have sat down and listened closely to your complaints. He would have focused intently on the description of your symptoms and upon his physical examination in order to make a diagnosis. Today doctors have little time to spend with a patient. In today's Health Maintenance Organization (HMO) environment, patients are herded in and out like cattle. After a brief visit, often lasting less than five minutes, the doctor will usually write a prescription for a drug that will only provide temporary relief of the primary complaint.

WORD WISE

Pharma. This root for both "pharmaceutical" and "pharmacy" refers broadly to drugs or medicine and has been used in the context of healing arts for several centuries. In its original Greek forms during antiquity, however, the word also had connotations of sorcery or even poison.

PHARMACEUTICAL FAILURE

Peggy's story typifies what is wrong with the current medical system and its primary method of treatment, which is simply to mask symptoms with harmful and toxic drugs or overuse antibiotics rather than build up the immune system. Mainstream medicine relies almost exclusively on pharmaceutical drugs to alleviate symptoms rather than searching for the underlying cause of declining health.

This type of polypharmacy is all too common and is destroying the lives of tens of millions of Americans.[8] Drugs are chemicals that never existed before in nature. They have been synthesized by the pharmaceutical companies and are administered to treat symptoms of diseases. As a matter of fact, all drugs must be detoxified by the liver. That means that drugs are toxins, which, according to *Merriam Webster's Dictionary*, are defined as poisons.

Medical doctors who still adhere to the current disease-model view of medicine believe that people can be made well through the use of pharmaceutical drugs rather than looking for the root cause of the patient's problems. Because of the massive advertising budgets of the drug companies, Americans have come to accept the notion that prescription drugs are the answer to their health woes.

No one is unhealthy or sick because they have low levels of pharmaceutical drugs in their body. Instead, health problems are caused by biochemical changes within our bodies that are commonly the result of poor nutrition, exposure to chemical pollutants or allergens, and the inevitable decline and imbalance of naturally occurring hormones as we age.

Yet our medicine cabinets are filled with drugs.

Are we healthier for it? One answer can be found in the educated individuals who are searching the Internet for alternative and natural solutions for their health problems[9] and abandoning traditional medicine by the millions. If medicine and drugs are the answer, why are so many Americans looking to alternative medicine? Perhaps it's because today's medicine is not providing a solution. You cannot poison yourself to good health, and the disease model of medicine, which offers drugs or surgery as a solution, has failed miserably to improve the health of many Americans.

DRUG DANGERS DOCUMENTED

You might think that I am overstating my position about the hazards of our reliance on pharmaceuticals, but an article entitled, "Incidence of Adverse Drug Reactions in Hospitalized Patients: A Meta-Analysis of Prospective Studies," published in the 1998 edition of the *Journal of the American Medical Association* (JAMA),[10] reported that *100,000 hospitalized patients die annually in America as a result of taking doctor-prescribed, FDA-approved drugs in the correct dosage.* That is equivalent to 725 Boeing 737 jet airplanes, fully loaded, crashing in one year. If that were to happen, there would be an outcry from Congress and the public. Another 750,000 Americans are seen in emergency rooms every year for treatment of adverse drug reactions.

SICK AND TIRED

This brings us to one of the key questions of this book: Are you sick and tired of being sick and tired? Another way of asking might be: Has your get-up-and-go got up and gone? Take a look at the statements below and see if any of them ring true in your experience:

- Your health is steadily deteriorating, yet your physician doesn't seem to be as concerned about it as you are.
- You've visited your doctor, complaining of extreme fatigue, weight gain, insomnia, mood swings, depressed moods, joint pain and muscle aches, brain fog, constipation, cold sensitivity, loss of libido, hair loss, or recurrent infections, only to be looked at as if you were a hypochondriac or neurotic.
- Your doctor has had your thyroid tested, only to tell you, "Your lab values are within the normal range." [11]

- Your doctor says that your symptoms are all a part of getting older.
- Your doctor has handed you samples of antidepressants as if you were some sort of psychiatric case.
- You're beginning to agree with your doctor that your symptoms may all be in your head.

If even half of these statements sound familiar to you, there's a good chance your deteriorating health is due to hypothyroidism. But you'll be relieved to know that there are solutions for you that can put you onto a path of health and wellness without the need to take pharmaceutical drugs that, at best, may only mask your symptoms and, at worst, may poison you.

A PERSONAL JOURNEY

Before delving into the subject of hypothyroidism, allow me to explain how I escaped the chains of conventional medicine to pursue natural approaches to health and wellness.

Between 1976 and 1988 I practiced medicine the way most physicians in this country do: I treated symptoms and diseases with drugs or surgery. When a patient came into my office with allergies, I prescribed an antihistamine. For a patient with high blood pressure, I prescribed an antihypertensive drug. If a patient suffered from joint pain, I prescribed an anti-inflammatory medication. There was an endless number of "antidotes" that I could prescribe to address one, some, or all of my patients' symptoms. When the drugs I prescribed had bothersome side effects, other drugs could be offered to take care of these additional symptoms.

For an acute illness, such as strep throat, sinus infection, or bronchitis, the drug approach, using antibiotics, is appropriate.

However, few patients with chronic ailments ever really get well using the drug approach. How can they? As I previously explained, chronic illness and disease are not caused by deficiencies of prescription drugs. The causes are complex, relating to poor nutrition, lack of exercise, a stressful lifestyle, a weakened immune system, and declines in levels of hormones, to name only a few of the key contributing factors.

By the time I reached my thirteenth year as a practicing physician, I had lost my passion for my chosen profession. I knew that the drugs I was prescribing for my patients' health problems were not making them feel better. Instead, in most cases, the drugs made them feel worse. However, prescribing drugs is what I had been taught to do. In truth, I was sick and tired of my patients always being sick and tired and so were they. I simply didn't know any other way to help my patients.

It was at this point that I began to seriously consider finding a new way to support my wife and eight children. What good was I doing? My patients weren't getting any better. At this crucial juncture, I was seriously considering abandoning my profession, but through God's divine providence, that was not to be. In 1989 I attended a medical conference on allergies and had the fortunate experience of hearing numerous physicians present cases about individuals who had the same problems as my patients. The difference was that their patients improved because they were addressing the underlying causes of disease. This was in stark contrast to what I had experienced with the patients in my practice.

By the time I reached my thirteenth year as a practicing physician, I had lost my passion for practicing medicine. I knew that the drugs I was prescribing for my patients' health problems were not making them feel better.

43

ENCOUNTERING HYPOTHYROIDISM

This conference inspired me to seek training in the diagnosis and treatment of allergies. Although I didn't know it at the time, this was the beginning of a new phase of my career. From that point onward, medicine became an immensely gratifying vocation for me because I found that I was able to get to the root causes of my patients' illnesses and enable them to obtain and maintain optimal health.

While traditional medicine focuses on treating symptoms rather than discovering and treating the underlying causes of the problems, I decided to take a different route and approach health and wellness from a natural perspective. What initially began as an allergy treatment program eventually evolved into our current eight-point treatment regimen. The backbone of this program is the treatment of hypothyroidism using desiccated thyroid hormone supplementation when indicated.

Before I entered the field of allergy medicine, I thought that hypothyroidism was a relatively rare condition in the United States. The introduction of iodized salt in the 1920s had virtually eliminated iodine deficiency as a major cause of hypothyroidism. In my 16-year career as a physician, I had seen only one case of myxedema, end-stage hypothyroidism, and that was during my internship at St. Joseph's Hospital in Houston in 1976. Myxedema takes years to develop and most patients with hypothyroidism are identified and treated long before this late stage occurs. The patient I saw during my internship had inexplicably gone without medical care until his condition was so severe that he required hospitalization. My medical mentor, Dr. Herb Fred, was able to diagnose this patient simply by looking at him. One day, while I was on duty, I was called to this patient's room by his frantic wife because he had quit breathing. I had to insert a breathing tube into his windpipe and attach the tube to a ventilator.

He was then transferred to the intensive care unit where the chief resident, Dr. Charles Butler, gave him intravenous thyroid hormone. Despite this frightening episode and the severity of this patient's condition, he made a remarkable recovery. In fact, five days after his near-death experience, he was chasing a nurse around his hospital room. This made a lasting impression on me as to the importance of the thyroid gland.

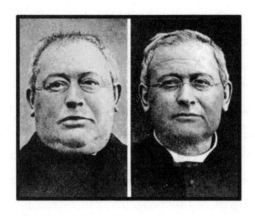

Historical patient before and after treatment for myxedema
Source: Hertoghe, E. Medical Record, Sep. 1914, Vol.86, Issue 12, 489-505.

Fast forward 16 years to March, 1992. At that time Dr. Richard Mabray, a successful obstetrician and gynecologist and a colleague of mine in the Pan American Allergy Society, encouraged me to evaluate my patients for autoimmune thyroiditis and hypothyroidism. He told me that I would be surprised by how many patients suffered with this disorder but had never been diagnosed or treated for it. Dr. Mabray also advised me to read *Hypothyroidism: The Unsuspected Illness* by Broda Barnes, MD. I did, and the insights that I gained from Dr. Barnes' book changed not only my life but also the lives of thousands of patients whom I have treated for hypothyroidism.

A CHANGE IN APPROACH

Since 1992 I and the other physicians at the Hotze Health & Wellness Center have treated more than 25,000 patients who have had the clinical symptoms of hypothyroidism with natural desiccated thyroid preparations such as Armour Thyroid, Nature-Throid, Westhroid, and compounded desiccated thyroid. Nothing can be more gratifying for a physician than to have his patients improve, get off their pharmaceutical drugs, and get their lives back. This was an uncommon occurrence when I practiced traditional medicine.

This natural approach offers a path to wellness through a diagnosis based upon your clinical history, coupled with the physician's observations and physical examinations. The treatment program relies on natural forms of thyroid, bioidentical hormone supplementation, treatment of yeast, as well as an optimal eating program, vitamin supplementation, and treatment of food and airborne allergies when indicated. The goal of this program is to increase your energy and strengthen your immune system. Physicians engage our guests in a transformative conversation by asking questions and taking time to listen their answers, rather than relying solely on laboratory tests for diagnosing and treating illness. This is a lost art in medicine.

Over the years, I continued to learn about new therapies that I could offer in order to provide better care for my guests. Although it happened gradually, medical thinking, heavily dependent upon pharmaceuticals and surgery, lost its grip on me. With a renewed purpose of my vocation, I began approaching health and wellness from a natural perspective. As my thinking changed, so did the suggestions that I offered my guests. As they implemented my recommendations, their health improved. They began to experience good health and a sense of wellness. Frequently, they would write or say to me in person the most gratifying words a doctor can hear from a patient, words no one had ever said to me when I was practicing traditional medicine: "Thank you for giving me my life back!"

──── WORD WISE ────

Guests. You have probably noticed that I use the term *guests* when writing about our patients. Our patients are our special, invited guests. They are welcomed with open arms and hearts filled with a desire to serve them and partner with them in order to help them restore their health, transform their lives, and improve their worlds, naturally. Shouldn't it be this way for everyone who visits a physician?

A WELLNESS PLAN

Thousands of men and women like Peggy have experienced repeated struggles with traditional treatments that didn't work and have come to our center to be evaluated. When our guests begin their journey onto the path of health and wellness, their progress is monitored based upon the resolution of their symptoms, not the results of a lab test. What good is a lab test that tells the doctor that you are normal when you know that you do not feel normal or well? Who should the doctor believe, you or the lab value? Hormonal declines and imbalances rarely demonstrate themselves on blood tests. The reason for this will be explained in a later chapter.

When our guests get well, they let us know it. If they are not improving, they also let us know! By listening to our guests, we are able to determine any adjustments that need to be made in their treatment program. Although the topic in this book is hypothyroidism, it is important for you to understand that the key to your health doesn't lie in placing just one piece in the puzzle.

My decision to educate you about hypothyroidism arises from my conviction that hypothyroidism has gone largely unrecognized and undiagnosed in America, yet it is the root cause of most common health problems.[12] The components of our comprehensive eight-point treatment program are as follows:

1. Treatment of low thyroid function can improve your energy, mood, memory and immune system, as well as restore feelings of well-being, just to name a few of the benefits.

2. Natural, bioidentical hormone replacement in men and women, especially in midlife when your hormones naturally decline, is a vital treatment because of the dramatic health improvements you will experience with balanced hormones.

3. Treatment of adrenal fatigue can also increase your vitality, immune system, and mental clarity.

4. Treatment of candida or yeast overgrowth can correct your digestive issues and weakened immune system.

5. A nutritionally balanced eating program will enable you to obtain and maintain an ideal body weight, which will prevent many diseases of aging and increase your life span.

6. Vitamin and mineral supplementation in large doses have been shown in thousands of studies to reduce your risk of developing diabetes, high blood pressure, heart disease, cancer, degenerative arthritis, obesity, and many other ailments.

7. Treatment of airborne allergies can strengthen your immune system and resolve your recurrent sinus and respiratory infections and asthma.

8. Treatment of food allergies can strengthen your immune system, heal your digestive system, and eradicate skin problems.

HYPOTHYROIDISM AND POLYPHARMACY: TWO HOT TOPICS

Without question, the most common hormonal issue is caused by low thyroid within the cells, or hypothyroidism. We are experiencing a silent, unrecognized global epidemic, which is especially prevalent in the United States.[13] According to recent studies, based upon blood tests alone, there are nearly 30 million Americans suffering from undiagnosed hypothyroidism.[14] If you were to base the diagnosis of hypothyroidism on clinical symptoms, physical findings, and low body temperature, there are upwards of approximately 100 million people plagued with this condition. These individuals are needlessly suffering from hypothyroid symptoms, such as debilitating fatigue, weight gain, insomnia, depression, joint and muscle pain, brain fog, loss of libido, constipation, cold sensitivity, recurrent infections, hair loss, infertility, and miscarriages, among many others.

We may be living longer, but have we really improved the quality of our lives? Americans are experiencing six rampant ailments: overweight/obesity, diabetes, hypertension, heart disease, degenerative arthritis, and cancer. These conditions inevitably lead to polypharmacy: the taking of a host of drugs.[15] According to a recent report, *18 to 20 percent of Americans spend their last days in an ICU, and despite most Americans' wish to spend their last days at home with family, 75 percent die in a hospital or a nursing home.*[16] These are sobering statistics that affect all of us. It is time for a change in mainstream medicine's current disease-care model to an approach of obtaining and maintaining health and wellness naturally.

A CALL TO ACTION

Our medical care should be determined by results rather than by manipulated research studies prepared by the pharmaceutical companies in order to market their new drugs to doctors and to the public on television commercials. Physicians should be held accountable by patients for their results. If you are not getting better under the care of your doctor, it's time for you to make a change.

Shouldn't you set a goal for yourself to become healthy and well? If you achieved this goal, would this enable you to tackle life head on and be successful in whatever endeavor you choose, whether you are a small business owner, an engineer, a teacher, a mother, or even a doctor? A healthy thyroid function is critical to your success. Yet, hypothyroidism commonly goes unrecognized or misdiagnosed by most medical doctors.

Because they feel that they are not being properly diagnosed, millions of people are dissatisfied with their medical care and are taking charge of their health. Most of our guests have come to us because they knew that something was wrong, despite their doctor's insistence that everything was normal.

The purpose of this book is to help you obtain and maintain health and wellness naturally so that you can enjoy a better quality of life. It will explain to you the underlying cause of these common symptoms and the actions that you can take to resolve them, based upon the success stories that the guests of the Hotze Health & Wellness Center have experienced.

It excites me to be able to share with you what I have learned and benefited from on my journey to find natural approaches to achieving a healthy life. This book will provide you with a solid foundation so that you too can achieve health and wellness naturally.

Are you ready to step outside the box and onto a path of health and wellness? Well then, let's get started.

SUMMARY

1. Today's medicine tries to alleviate symptoms but does not address the root causes of a person's medical problems.

2. Pharmaceutical drugs are the default button of medical treatment even though they are toxins that cause wide-ranging side effects.

3. The disease model and its emphasis on drug treatment have not stemmed the tide of problems affecting large segments of the population.

4. A natural approach to treatment produces superior results, especially for the wide range of common symptoms associated with hypothyroidism.

5. For more information, please visit www.hotzehwc.com/Hypothyroidism.

chapter
TWO

THE UNDIAGNOSED ILLNESS

TERRI'S STORY

"They told me I had Alzheimer's."

If you were to describe someone who was a go-getter, full of energy, and always involved in a flurry of activities, you would have been describing Terri. Terri and Pat, her husband of 20 years, had fostered 23 children and adopted five others. Not having enough to do to occupy her time, Terri had started and developed her own successful business of training youths in gymnastics. To say that she was a busy woman would be an understatement.

During this time, Terri experienced five miscarriages before finally giving birth to her only biological son. It was during her last pregnancy at age 30 that Terri developed complications that led to her being hospitalized for eight weeks prior to delivery. Her doctor could not determine why she was constantly nauseous and throwing up, leaving her weak from dehydration. She felt as if she had a severe case of the flu, not for a few days but for the entire nine months of her pregnancy. Additional specialists and even a psychiatrist evaluated

Terri in an attempt to discover the cause of her condition. Eventually her physician told her, "Your problems are all in your head." When she heard this, Terri became livid and shouted at the doctor. She told him that she was not mentally imbalanced, and that she didn't dream up her nausea to the point of dehydration, just to get her doctors' attention. But the doctors wouldn't listen to her. This was the beginning of the decline in her health.

ONGOING DECLINE

After the birth of her son, Terri's health plummeted. She was then in her early 30s, and her periods felt like the onset of the flu and were also associated with migraines, bloating, and cramps. Instead of being able to enjoy her new baby, Terri was afflicted with recurrent sinus infections, bronchitis, asthma, allergies, and sensitivity to chemicals such as smoke and perfumes. Terri's chronic infections led her to take one antibiotic after another. She was burning the candle at both ends, trying to be a supportive wife and mother, and still maintain a successful business. Fatigue was a byword. Over the next 13 years, despite her poor health, Terri somehow managed to keep all the balls she was juggling in the air.

Finally, Terri lost the grip on her life. Despite being exhausted during the day, she could not sleep for more than two hours at a time. Her extreme fatigue left her unable to manage her family and business obligations. It took every ounce of strength and energy she possessed just to get out of bed. In addition, she had lost all desire for sexual intimacy. She began steadily gaining weight, her complexion worsened, and her hair began to fall out. Terri did not even have the energy or desire to wear makeup or improve her appearance. She became unmotivated and irritable. The joints in her hands were so stiff that signing payroll checks became a painful chore.

Terri was hesitant to see a doctor about her symptoms because of the dismissive way she had been treated in the past. Her husband, children, employees, and mother began to recognize that her health and mental status were deteriorating, and they expressed their concerns.

Terri lost her mental sharpness and started to have difficulty remembering specific words. She experienced frightening lapses in memory in which she could not even remember what the inside of her company's building looked like, even though she had designed it. It was this significant memory loss that led her family to insist that she be evaluated by her physician.

MULTIPLE MISDIAGNOSES

At first her doctor prescribed birth control pills that only made matters worse.

Another physician diagnosed Terri with depression and recommended that she take antidepressants. Terri thought, "Okay, he says I'm depressed, but what am I depressed about?" She had no reason to be depressed. She had a wonderful husband and family and a successful business. Terri thought, "I am not depressed. I am just exhausted." She submitted to test after test, but no answers were forthcoming. The doctors' only solutions were to mask the symptoms with drugs.

As a last resort, Terri was evaluated by a specialist in Alzheimer's disease at Baylor College of Medicine in Houston, and was told that she had Alzheimer's. Terri was just 43 years of age.

Then one Sunday morning, while she lay on the couch in front of the television, Terri received a small glimmer of hope as she watched an interview with a vibrant woman who spoke enthusiastically about how she had regained her health. The speaker was television celebrity Suzanne Somers, describing her own long road back to health and wellness, and sharing the stories of other women who had taken a similar path in dealing with hypothyroidism. As Terri listened, the stories eerily reminded her of her own story except, with her, there had been no happy ending. She prayed to God for help and direction.

FINDING THE ROAD TO WELLNESS

When Terri came to the Hotze Health & Wellness Center, after learning that we treated hypothyroidism, her evaluation with Don Ellsworth, MD was the first time she felt that a doctor had listened to her and understood her problems. She was prescribed natural desiccated thyroid as one point of her regimen, as well as bioidentical female hormones.

Within the first month Terri began to notice significant improvement. The nausea, bloating, migraines, mood swings, and flu-like symptoms associated with her menstrual cycle resolved. Over the next four weeks, she experienced steady weight loss without having to exercise. Now she was finally sleeping soundly and could actually carry on a conversation without losing her train of thought. Her energy level markedly increased so that she was able to return to church and participate in other social activities. She felt so good that she hired a personal trainer and began working out with her husband three days a week. By the third month, she had lost 15 pounds and felt mentally sharp. Her hair was healthier, her complexion had cleared, and she was sleeping restfully without having to take sleep medication. She even added tennis to her weekly schedule.

SIGNS OF A TROUBLED MEDICAL SYSTEM

If you're worried about becoming overweight or developing high blood pressure, diabetes, heart disease, cancer, or degenerative arthritis, you should be because the statistics for these diseases among Americans are sobering:

- Heart disease is the number-one killer, leading to the death of more than 750,000 Americans each year, evenly divided between men and women.
- More than 550,000 will succumb to cancer this year.
- Type 2 diabetes, formerly named adult onset diabetes, will be diagnosed in 23 million adults this year alone.
- One-third of all adult Americans have high blood pressure.
- There were 750,000 joint replacements in 2007. By 2015 this number will rise to 2,000,000 joint replacements.
- More than 100,000 individuals will die annually from the adverse effects of legally prescribed, FDA-approved drugs.

In the current medical paradigm, both patients and their doctors are attempting to repair damage that has already occurred.

A GROWING EPIDEMIC

Terri's plight is common. Undiagnosed hypothyroidism affects tens of millions of people in the United States. As we saw in Chapter 1, even conventional medicine estimates—based on blood tests alone—that nearly 30 million Americans are suffering from undiagnosed hypothyroidism and the range of symptoms it includes.

With all the advances in modern medicine, you would have thought that the riddle of illness caused by hypothyroidism would have been solved. We can diagnose and monitor an astronaut's health condition in space, yet millions of Americans walk into their doctor's office with symptoms of hypothyroidism and are dismissed as depressed hypochondriacs. As outlined in Chapter 1, their blood tests are pronounced "normal," and instead of being given a therapeutic trial of natural desiccated thyroid, they are given a prescription for antidepressants, antianxiety drugs, anti-inflammatory drugs, or sleep medication to mask their symptoms, as well as an admonition that they need to "Learn to live with it. It's part of getting older."

I'm often asked the question, "Why doesn't my doctor understand?" I have strong opinions about this as I am convinced there remains a place for good, old-fashioned, common-sense medicine. Many doctors have traded the art of medicine for a "paint-by-number" treatment. By trying to diagnose the cause of symptoms based upon blood tests alone, doctors are neglecting the most important pieces of the clinical puzzle: your symptoms, history, physical condition, and low body temperature[17].

You may have watched your parents or grandparents age in a less than graceful fashion from years of overmedication, leaving them a shell of the people that they once were, spending their last days in a nursing home or hospital.

This downhill course does not have to be inevitable. You can resolve the symptoms of hypothyroidism. You can also dramatically lower your risk of obesity, high blood pressure, type 2 diabetes, heart disease, cancer, and degenerative arthritis, vastly improving the quality of your life. The second half of your life could actually be better than the first. Read on for a roadmap to better health.

WHY IS HYPOTHYROIDISM MORE
PREVALENT TODAY?

Do you ever wonder why there are so many more people suffering from illnesses such as heart disease, autoimmune disorders, degenerative diseases such as arthritis and osteoporosis, diabetes, cancer, and hypertension today than in the past? Of course, there have been changes in our diet and an increased exposure to toxins in our environment. But there is one other change that has occurred, making hypothyroidism more prevalent.

Hypothyroidism is often manifested by susceptibility to infections secondary to a weakened immune system. Prior to antibiotics, people with hypothyroidism often never survived childhood. Less than 150 years ago, half of all children died before reaching adulthood. The Captain of Death in the world prior to 1940 was tuberculosis.

Then, in the 1930s, lifesaving antibiotics were discovered. Antibiotics have enabled millions of people to escape early death from infections. We have always had two populations: those who were resistant to infection, with healthy thyroid function, and those with hypothyroidism who were more susceptible to diseases. The latter group was termed the "new population" by Dr. Broda Barnes, renowned physician and life-long researcher of hypothyroidism, whose work I referenced in Chapter 1. Because of antibiotics, this new population survived the infectious diseases that once ravaged the populations of the United States and European industrialized nations. Rather than dying of childhood infections, they began to survive into adulthood and have offspring of their own. Their life span has been lengthened, but their quality of life is impaired. This is one reason that symptoms of hypothyroidism are increasingly apparent in our population today. These individuals not only continue to suffer from the effects of hypothyroidism into adulthood, but, as Dr. Barnes hypothesized in his research, hypothyroid individuals, who would have previously perished from tuberculosis and other infectious diseases, are now dying of cardio-vascular diseases, diabetes, and cancer instead.

Unfortunately, hypothyroidism is largely overlooked, and those with hypothyroidism continue to struggle against illness and infection. These individuals need to be educated about how hypothyroidism can lead to a host of other health problems.

Prior to antibiotics, people with hypothyroidism often never survived childhood.

IT'S ALL IN YOUR THROAT

The name thyroid is derived from the Greek word *thyreoeides*, which means "shield." The thyroid gland is located in the front of your neck below the trachea or Adam's apple and is, to some eyes, indeed shaped like a shield. Others note that the gland is more the shape and size of a monarch butterfly. However you view the gland, it controls your body's metabolism. Metabolism means the sum of the physical and chemical processes in your cells that produce material and energy so that your body can function.

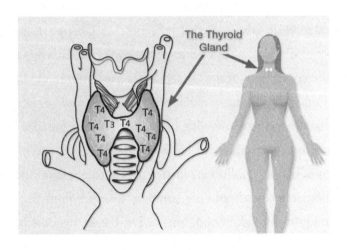

The Thyroid Gland

Though you may think of the food you eat as a source of your energy, your body requires more than food to build and maintain itself. The energy currency inside your body is a molecule called adenosine triphosphate (ATP). Your cells generate ATP from glucose through a complex series of chemical reactions that require the presence of thyroid hormones.

SPARK PLUG FOR THE BODY

When you put gasoline in your car's gas tank, this simple act is not sufficient to make your car run. The gasoline must flow through the fuel line and into the engine's combustion chamber. Inside the combustion chamber, the spark plugs must give off a spark to rupture the bonds between the gasoline molecules, which releases energy. This energy then drives the pistons, making the car run. Excess energy is expelled through the tailpipe as heat.

In your body, thyroid hormone functions as the spark plug of the cell. It causes the combustion of glucose, converting the energy stored within its bonds into ATP, which fuels the cellular reactions that keep your body humming along. Instead of being expelled, excess energy that's generated as heat keeps your body warm.

If you have an eight-cylinder car, but only seven spark plugs are working, your car will run, but it will run rough and not perform optimally. In the same way, if your cells do not have adequate levels of thyroid hormone, the energy contained in the glucose molecule will not efficiently convert to ATP, the energy molecule of the cell. The result will be decreased energy and lowered metabolism. If your thyroid gland were removed, your body would wind down like a toy soldier and cease to function altogether. Without thyroid replacement therapy, you would be dead within a year or two.

TWO THYROID HORMONES

Other than surgical removal of the thyroid gland, there are two primary causes for a decline in the cells' supply of thyroid hormones:

1. Inadequate production of thyroid hormones by the thyroid gland
2. Inadequate absorption of thyroid hormones by the cells

We're going to look at these two problems in greater detail in a moment. But first, let's clarify: I have been speaking of thyroid hormone as if it were a single hormone, but there are actually two.

The thyroid gland produces a protein called thyroglobulin, and iodine atoms attach to this protein to make the thyroid hormones. These two primary thyroid hormones are:

- thyroxine, known as T4, which has four (4) iodine atoms
- triiodothyronine, known as T3, which has three (3) iodine atoms

Chemically speaking, the two hormones look almost identical except for the number of iodine atoms they contain. But the thyroid gland produces them in different amounts. Approximately 93 percent of the gland's thyroid hormone production is in the form of T4, and the remaining 7 percent is in the form of T3. Despite its higher level of production within the thyroid gland, T4 is the inactive form of the thyroid hormone. T3 is the active thyroid hormone. Only T3—or T4 that has been converted into T3 within the cells of your body— can be used to produce energy in our cells. This distinction is very important, as we'll see.

IMAGE OF T3 AND T4 HORMONES

Triiodothyronine (T3)

Thyroxine (T4)

In other words, to produce the additional T3 needed for proper thyroid hormone function within your cells, your body converts T4 to T3, thanks to an enzyme called deiodinase, which cleaves an iodine atom off the T4 molecule to make T3. Not only does this conversion occur in your individual cells but also in both the liver and the intestines. This underscores the importance of maintaining a healthy liver and gastrointestinal system in order for you to have adequate T3 available for your cells.

HUMMING HEALTHY HORMONES

It is through the secretion of thyroid hormones that the thyroid gland controls your metabolism. The thyroid hormones are then released into your blood stream, which carries them to the trillions of cells in your body. In the cells, thyroid hormones produce energy by stimulating the mitochondria, which are the energy factories inside your cells that produce the energy and heat necessary for life.

Your body needs energy to function just as a car needs the energy from the combustion of gasoline to run the engine. When your thyroid gland is producing adequate amounts of thyroid hormones and these hormones are being properly utilized by your cells, you have energy and vitality. Your immune system is so strong that you have resistance to infections. You are able to naturally balance your weight, think clearly, feel alert, and enthusiastically embrace the day knowing that you will have enough energy to get your work done without being exhausted. The excess energy production of the cells is given off as heat to ensure that the body operates at the most efficient temperature.

Your metabolism depends upon the healthy production of thyroid hormones and the proper utilization of these hormones by the cells. In addition to affecting your weight, thyroid hormones are important for the production of human growth hormone, control of sugar levels, proper bone growth, strong muscles, a healthy immune system, normal heart rhythm and circulation, proper digestion and bowel function, and healthy sleep patterns. Every cell in your body requires thyroid hormones for energy. Most importantly, the thyroid hormone affects energy production in your brain, which requires 20 percent of the energy production of your entire body.

The thyroid also partners with other hormones to insure that your body functions optimally as you age. This is one of the main reasons that Terri responded so quickly and so well to the treatment program prescribed for her at the Hotze Health & Wellness Center. It was a comprehensive program that included not just thyroid supplementation, but several other natural bioidentical hormones and supplements that her body lacked in sufficient amounts to maintain vibrant health. In a coming chapter, the topic of bioidentical hormones will be discussed in more detail. The bottom line is that thyroid hormone is essential for a healthy, productive life.

WHEN THYROID HORMONES FALTER

Since having adequate thyroid hormone ensures proper function of many bodily functions, lack of thyroid hormone causes problems that are just as wide-ranging. Among the manifestations:

- As we age, all our hormone levels decline, including thyroid. This decline and imbalance in our naturally occurring hormones adversely affects thyroid hormone function and metabolism within our cells.
- A sluggish metabolism from hypothyroidism leads to an inability to properly burn fat and lose weight. Weight loss is difficult for hypothyroid individuals even when they lower their caloric intake.
- Your body functions best at 98.6 degrees Fahrenheit, but hypothyroid patients have temperatures that are 97 or 96 or lower. This is why many hypothyroid individuals are sensitive to the cold—their bodies cannot generate enough energy and heat to keep them warm.
- Because the brain takes so much energy, hypothyroid individuals tend to experience a decline in their mental sharpness—the "brain fog" that so many patients describe.

THE THYROID FEEDBACK SYSTEM

It will be helpful for you to understand something called the thyroid feedback system, which works much like the thermostat in your home. The thermostat senses when to adjust the temperature. For optimal thyroid function, the thyroid gland enlists two lieutenants as thermostats: the hypothalamus and the pituitary gland, both located in your brain.

The hypothalamus is located above the brain stem at the base of the brain, monitoring and responding to what is occurring inside your body as well as external factors such as heat, cold, and stress. When it senses stressors or pressures, the hypothalamus knows that your body needs to adjust and sends thyrotropin-releasing hormone (TRH) to the pituitary gland. TRH acts like a chemical Paul Revere, readying the pituitary gland to send its own messenger to the thyroid gland.

In response to the rallying cry of TRH, the pituitary sends thyroid-stimulating hormone (TSH) to the thyroid gland to signal the need for production and release of more thyroid hormones. Your pituitary—a small, peanut-sized gland in the brain—also monitors thyroid level fluctuations in the blood. A properly functioning pituitary gland senses that thyroid hormone levels are low in the blood and releases TSH of its own accord, commanding the production of thyroid hormone.

Thyroid hormones are then released into the bloodstream where they become messengers themselves, traveling to each organ to give individualized instructions to the cells on how to operate. Without adequate amounts of thyroid hormones, the cells and organs of your body operate sluggishly. This is why the symptoms of hypothyroidism are so varied—to the point that they can seem disconnected from one another.

In summary, your body has two checkpoints, the hypothalamus and pituitary, to assure that it is producing adequate amounts of thyroid. This feedback system is important to understand because it has bearing on current laboratory tests that are used to diagnose hypothyroidism. These laboratory tests will be discussed in a later chapter.

This brings up an interesting point. We have several ways to measure the thyroid hormone level in your blood, but no blood test to actually determine how much active thyroid hormone you have within your cells. That would be helpful to know, as we'll see by taking a look at the effect that thyroid hormones have within your cells.

WHAT'S HAPPENING IN YOUR CELLS?

A quick review: There are two main thyroid hormones, thyroxine, also called T4, and triiodothyronine, or T3.

T3 is the active hormone—it possesses four times the activity of T4.

T4 is the inactive hormone—it must be converted into T3 inside the cell before it can be used.

The numbers 3 and 4 refer to the number of iodine atoms that are attached to the hormone. T4 has four iodine atoms and T3 has three iodine atoms.

As T4 enters a cell, a specific enzyme removes one of its iodine atoms turning it into T3, the active hormone.

Most doctors often assume that every bit of the thyroid hormone in the blood is being received properly by your cells and that it is being converted from T4, the inactive hormone, into T3, the active hormone. This would be a correct assumption if we lived in a perfect world, but we don't.

Think of it this way: Imagine firewood neatly stacked on the hearth next to the fireplace. It's there and it's ready to be burned, but if someone doesn't pick it up and put it into the flames of the fireplace, it won't burn. This is analogous to the way that thyroid hormone works. You may have an adequate amount of thyroid hormone in your blood indicating a picture-perfect lab result, but if thyroid hormones are not actually being assimilated into your cells in adequate amounts, you will not receive the full benefit.

Synthetic thyroid medications such as Synthroid and Levoxyl contain only T4, the inactive thyroid. It then must be converted to T3, the active form of the hormone, once it gets into the cells of the body. Many individuals do not efficiently make that conversion. This is one reason why natural desiccated thyroid preparations containing T3, such as Armour Thyroid, Nature-Throid, and Hotze thyroid (desiccated thyroid USP compounded at the Hotze Pharmacy), work much better than their synthetic counterparts that contain only T4. (The term *desiccated* simply means "dried.")

It has been my experience in treating more than 25,000 patients with natural desiccated thyroid that desiccated thyroid hormone is the best treatment for hypothyroidism. I remember asking one of my mentors, Dr. Dor Brown, in 1992, why he thought I should use Armour Thyroid, which is a desiccated thyroid hormone product, rather than the more commonly prescribed Synthroid. He simply and emphatically stated, "It works!" Sometimes, simple is best.

> *Synthetic thyroid medications contain only T4,*
> *the inactive thyroid.*

THE REST OF TERRI'S STORY

Terri's low thyroid function was one of the root causes of many of the various debilitating symptoms that she had been enduring. For her, supplementation with desiccated thyroid was life changing. In addition to regaining her health and vitality, something happened that was quite remarkable. Four months after coming to our center,

Terri was feeling so good that, at her children's prompting, she decided to enter the Mrs. Texas United States Pageant in 2006 and won! She went on to win the title of Mrs. United States of America the following year. This never would have happened if she had not been diagnosed and treated for hypothyroidism.

A SIMPLE TEST

If your thyroid hormones are not functioning properly at the cellular level, you may experience the symptoms of hypothyroidism. There is not a blood test to measure how much active thyroid hormone is actually being utilized in your cells, but there is a simple test that you can perform at home or work to determine your metabolism: Just place a thermometer in your mouth and measure your body temperature. It should be 98.6. If it is one or two degrees below that, you have low energy production in your cells and likely have hypothyroidism, especially if you are experiencing many of the diverse symptoms of hypothyroidism.

SUMMARY

1. Millions suffer from hypothyroidism, yet their condition is often misdiagnosed or overlooked in a medical system that places more emphasis on prescribing drugs.
2. Your thyroid gland controls your metabolism and regulates a wide range of bodily functions from weight control and body heat to mental sharpness and a healthy immune system.
3. Your thyroid gland needs both T3 and T4 thyroid hormones to operate at an optimal level. The more abundant T4 can convert to T3, the active form, but doesn't always do so efficiently.

4. The brain's hypothalamus and pituitary gland help monitor the body and stimulate production of thyroid hormones when needed.

5. Synthetic thyroid is not a sufficient substitute for thyroid supplementation because it only contains T4.

6. You may have "normal" levels of thyroid hormones in your blood and "pass" blood tests, but that does not mean those thyroid hormones are being converted properly into your cells.

7. For more information, please visit www.hotzehwc.com/Wellness101/Hypothyroidism.

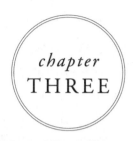

chapter
THREE

SYMPTOMS AND DIAGNOSIS

LAURIE'S STORY

"I felt like life was passing me by. I was missing out on my children's lives because when I was there, I was never really there."

When she first visited us at the Hotze Health & Wellness Center, Laurie was a 29-year-old mother of two small children. Her recently established business was thriving. She had the beautiful family that she had always hoped for, and the fulfillment of a life-long dream of becoming an entrepreneur, yet she found that she was not able to enjoy her success because of her developing health issues.

Laurie felt as if she were sitting in front of a black and white television watching her own life pass by in slow motion, void of color, just hues of gray. Her brain was constantly in a fog. It was more than just being scatterbrained. To be able to concentrate and focus required all her energy. The brain fog never lifted and her thoughts were not clear or concise. Her daily short-term memory loss and muddled thinking had become either the brunt of jokes or the source of aggravation to those around her. She had to laugh at herself because that's all she could do, but it was becoming increasingly embarrassing. She was fatigued to the point of exhaustion, and she found herself becoming irritated at the most minor incidences.

AN EARLY DIAGNOSIS

In her early twenties, Laurie had been diagnosed with hypo-thyroidism and had been treated with Synthroid, a preparation that contains only T4, the inactive thyroid prohormone. Despite the fact that her doctor did not inspire confidence in her regarding his ability to regulate her hypothyroidism, Laurie was a "good patient" and followed his recommendations. The medication made her feel slightly better, but not well. Laurie was determined to pull herself up by the bootstraps and just get on with her life.

After the birth of her second child, it was apparent that all the positive thinking and willpower she could muster was not going to enable her to get her health back. She just could not fake it anymore. The brain fog, memory loss, PMS, allergies, chronic exhaustion, stomach problems, hair loss, anxiety, and insomnia were just too much for her to overcome on her own. She coveted sleep and obses-sively counted the hours she could get before she had to wake up each morning. Laurie told her husband that the only thing she wanted for her birthday was a night at a hotel, to sleep alone.

Laurie could handle being embarrassed in social situations, but it was beginning to affect her family. Her fatigue was so bad that at one point Laurie fell asleep while feeding her baby in his high chair and woke up 30 minutes later. She would nod off while reading to her boys and give her toddler empty answers to his questions because she didn't have enough energy to engage. Laurie told me that she could tell that her toddler wondered why Mommy couldn't play anymore. Laurie wondered the same thing. It was breaking her heart to think of all she was missing. She was trying her best, but she just couldn't be the mom and wife that she so desired to be.

When she did visit her obstetrician for a follow up appointment, she was embarrassed to tell her everything that was going on so she just hit the high points. Even so, Laurie was shocked when her physician's solution was to prescribe her an antidepressant. She found this recommendation odd because she had not said anything about feeling depressed, only that she was sick and tired of feeling sick and tired. Refusing the antidepressant prescription, Laurie did what many other women have done; she put a smile on her face and kept going with grit and determination despite her debilitating symptoms.

Laurie began thinking that she must be dying from a terminal illness and that it was going to be discovered too late. If she were terminally ill, she would rather be given a diagnosis so that she could accept it and make arrangements for whatever amount of time she had left. Worse yet, it scared her to think that if this was what life was like at 29, what would it be like at 40 or 50? She felt isolated. She knew that she didn't deserve this, and neither did her children or husband. This is when Laurie decided to take charge of her health. She was convinced that if she searched hard and long enough that she would find a solution.

VAST IMPROVEMENT

Laurie came to us after reading about our evaluation and treatment program in my first book, *Hormones, Health, and Happiness*. At first, she was hesitant to describe her symptoms to Dr. Ellsworth because of her experiences with other physicians, who had been dismissive and condescending. But Dr. Ellsworth listened and explained how common her symptoms were. Instead of antidepressants, he prescribed a treatment program consisting of natural desiccated thyroid, bioidentical sex hormones, adrenal support, vitamin and mineral supplementation, and a yeast-free eating plan.

Almost immediately after her initial appointment, Laurie's brain fog lifted. Instead of feeling as if she were teetering on the precipice of disaster, she woke up feeling alive. Throughout the rest of the day, she waited for her symptoms to show up and prepared herself for the afternoon "slump hour." The slump never came, nothing hurt, and she sailed through the afternoon with energy. She called her friends and family to tell them how fantastic she felt. Instead of watching her life on a black and white television, she felt as if she were living in Technicolor. Instead of standing outside, watching her life pass by, she was actually living it. She no longer counts the hours of sleep before it's time for her to wake up. With her vitality and zest for life restored, and her symptoms a distant memory, Laurie can't wait to get up and get after it every day!

COULD YOU HAVE HYPOTHYROIDISM?

Do Laurie's symptoms and story resonate with you? Laurie's history is similar to the stories of most of the 25,000-plus guests who have sought solutions at the Hotze Health & Wellness Center. They have had a host of debilitating symptoms, and the only solutions offered by the medical world were drugs to mask their symptoms. Millions of Americans have no idea that their problems are related to a hypothyroid condition. So how can you know if hypothyroidism is affecting you? Surprisingly, the best place to begin is not with your blood test, but rather, with your medical history, your physical signs and symptoms, as well as the measurement of your body temperature.

Laurie was tested for hypothyroidism, and in her case, her blood tests indicated that she was indeed low in thyroid. But you may have been tested for thyroid on several occasions only to have your doctor dismiss your symptoms and say that your blood work was within the normal range. Because of my 23 years of clinical experience with more than 25,000 guests at our center, it is my conviction that, when guests present with multiple symptoms of hypothyroidism, even when their blood tests do not show a corresponding low level of thyroid hormone, they deserve a therapeutic trial of natural desiccated thyroid hormones. Unfortunately, there are too few physicians who share this view. Remember, thyroid hormones affect every cell of your body. They enable your cells to produce the energy needed to regulate tissue growth, keep your immune system healthy, and help to maintain blood pressure and fluid balance. Because thyroid hormones are required by every organ and cell in the body, when your cells lack adequate thyroid hormones, a wide range of seemingly unrelated symptoms develop.

SYMPTOMS AND SIGNS OF HYPOTHYROIDISM

Most people associate hypothyroidism with low energy and weight gain, but, as we have discussed, there are actually a host of other symptoms that can be caused by a low thyroid condition. Patients with low thyroid can experience anything from depression, headaches, joint and muscle pain, digestive disorders, and poor concentration to women's menstrual issues, and impaired fertility. If the deficiency is present during pregnancy, premature delivery, stillbirth, or miscarriages can occur. A patient may have one, some, or all of the following signs and symptoms depending upon the degree of hypothyroidism.

- fatigue
- difficulty with weight
- cold hands and feet

- low body temperature
- tingling and numbness in extremities
- problems with mental focus
- decline in mental sharpness; brain fog
- enlarged thyroid gland
- brittle fingernails with ridging
- insomnia
- mood swings
- depressed moods
- joint and muscle aches and pains
- irritable bowel syndrome
- sluggish bowel function/constipation
- headaches
- frequent infections
- irregular menstrual cycles
- infertility
- miscarriages
- loss of libido
- hair loss in females
- loss of the lateral third of the eyebrows
- enlarged tongue with indentations
- elevated cholesterol
- dry skin
- low blood pressure
- decreased sweating
- hoarseness
- pale or pasty complexion
- slow in speech
- prone to rambling
- fluid retention

- allergies

Hypothyroidism can reveal itself in one or more of any of these symptoms and the manifestation will vary from person to person. If you are experiencing any of these symptoms, you may benefit from a therapeutic trial of natural desiccated thyroid supplementation.

Following are illustrations of some of the classical features associated with low thyroid function, including a puffy face, ridging of the nails, swollen tongue, and hair loss.

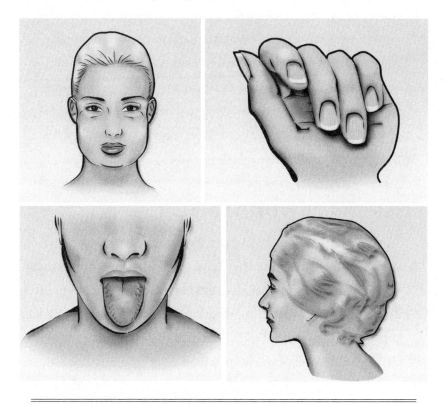

THE PROBLEM OF
DISPARAGING DOCTORS

Women's lives have been placed in jeopardy by the accepted medical view that looks no further than a prescription pad. This is a result of the condescending and dismissive attitude taken toward women's health complaints by the male-oriented medical community. Women are viewed as neurotics, hysterics, and hypochondriacs. Most physicians have little or no understanding of the adverse effects that are caused by hormonal decline and imbalance although they are confronted daily by women who describe their problems to them. If physicians understood the cause of these problems, they would be able to treat the root cause and resolve these women's symptoms. Instead, doctors load up women patients with psychiatric drugs. Many women have been incorrectly labeled "hypochondriacs" when their blood tests return normal. Yet normal blood tests don't stop physicians from prescribing women antianxiety drugs, antidepressants, or sleep medication. It grieves me to think of how many women have been mistreated by this type of medicine, with nothing to show for it but a cabinet full of drugs and their side effects, and often, ruined lives, marriages, relationships and self-esteem.

DIAGNOSING HYPOTHYROIDISM

A respected mentor during my days as an intern once told me: "A patient will tell you what they have if you simply listen to them." He was right; my patients began to get better when I started to listen. While blood tests can be an important tool, most doctors look exclusively at blood tests instead of listening to their patients.

If a physician relies solely on blood tests to determine whether or not a patient has hypothyroidism, what is the purpose of the office visit? Why not just draw the patient's blood for study and save the time, expense, and humiliation of an appointment? The single most important tool in determining a patient's thyroid function is for the physician to complete a thorough review of the patient's symptoms and history along with a physical examination that must include the patient's body temperature. Remember, a classical feature of hypo-thyroidism is a low body temperature. The healthy body temperature is 98.6. Temperatures that are 1 to 2 degrees below this are an indication of a low metabolism caused by hypothyroidism. Laboratory results can occasionally be helpful in confirming a diagnosis, but they do not trump the patient's signs and symptoms.

PATIENTS DON'T LIE; LAB TESTS DO.

It is difficult to get a diagnosis of hypothyroidism in the United States because current medicine chooses to view laboratory tests as the gold standard for diagnosing it. You may have every single symptom of low thyroid, but if your thyroid stimulating hormone (TSH) level is in the "normal" range, hypothyroidism will go undiagnosed.

Even though physicians use the TSH as the main test for diagnosing hypothyroidism, it does not measure the amount of thyroid hormone produced by your body. In fact, the TSH is not a hormone that is produced by the thyroid gland; rather, it is a pituitary gland hormone. Physicians focus on the TSH because when the pituitary gland is functioning normally, it is supposed to fluctuate up or down depending on how much thyroid hormone is in the blood.

Using blood tests as the sole determinant of whether you have hypothyroidism is faulty for the following reasons.

1. "Normal" values are arbitrary.

The range of the TSH that is considered "normal" is as wide as the Grand Canyon...

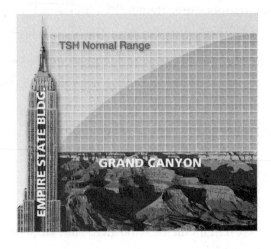

...and as tall as the Empire State building. It is important for you to understand how the "normal" lab range is defined. It is an arbitrary value chosen by the laboratory company that performs the blood testing, and is based upon the average results of the previous 1,000 patients studied for the same test. The normal range is then defined by the laboratory company as falling 47.5 percent below the average, or mean, and 47.5 percent above the average. Therefore, 95 percent of the population will always fall within the normal range. However, you can be certain that 95 percent of the population does not feel normal and full of energy. Nor do they feel healthy and well.

Just because your thyroid blood value falls within the so-called normal range, that does not mean that your thyroid hormones are at an optimal level for you or that they are being adequately used by your cells.

IF THE SHOE DOESN'T
FIT, DON'T WEAR IT

Think of walking into a shoe store looking for a size 7 pair of shoes. The clerk hands you a pair of shoes to try on. After walking in them for a minute, you return them to the clerk stating that your toes are crunched and your feet ache. You tell him the shoes are clearly too small. Instead of giving you a larger size, he tells you that the shoes are within the "normal range" of shoe sizes for the population and there is nothing wrong with the shoes; instead, there is something wrong with your thinking. Now you would find this clerk ridiculous, wouldn't you? Just as shoes are not one-size-fits-all, an optimal thyroid lab value for one person may not be an optimal level for another.

2. **Standards have changed over time.**

Between 1991 and 2012, the normal laboratory range for the free thyroxine (T4) blood test has been lowered by 15 percent, from 0.90–2.00ng/dl to 0.76–1.7ng/dl. What does this mean to you? If you had seen your physician in 1991 and had a free T4 value of 0.80ng/dl, you would have been classified as hypothyroid. However, if you visited your physician in 2012 with this same lab value, no diagnosis would have been made.

Why has this lowering of the thyroid hormone level by the laboratories occurred? As the baby boomers age, more and more of them are being tested for hypothyroidism, which skews the average score to a lower level. Healthy, young people do not routinely have their thyroid hormone levels checked. So the current laboratory range for thyroid is representative of the range for older people, not young, healthy people. Thyroid hormone levels and the utilization of thyroid hormone by the cells inevitably decline with age. This decline may be a normal part of the aging process, but it is not a healthy situation. So while you may be suffering from the symptoms of hypothyroidism, there is a 95 percent chance that your thyroid blood levels will fall within the wide range of "normal" and that your hypothyroid condition will remain undiagnosed.

3. Results don't match clinical experience.

My clinical experience with lab tests has also made me skeptical. The same blood samples from 40 of my patients were sent to two different labs for measurement of their thyroid levels, and their results varied by as much as 50 percent! Which lab test result am I going to believe? This is one key reason that I listen to my patients. I will always believe them before believing a lab test on hormones.

The lab test is a snapshot of what is going on in the blood at that moment in time. Circulating thyroid hormone levels in your blood vary throughout the day and are influenced by disease processes, prescription drugs, other hormones, environmental chemicals, and stressors.

> *The same blood samples from 40 of my patients were sent to two different labs for measurement of their thyroid levels and their results varied by as much as 50 percent!*

A BROKEN THERMOSTAT

As I mentioned in Chapter 2, your pituitary gland helps set your body's thermostat. It sends the message that your thyroid hormones need an adjustment. In order to boost thyroid hormone production, the pituitary gland produces more TSH when the thyroid gland is not producing enough thyroid hormone. Conversely, the pituitary gland secretes less TSH when the thyroid gland is producing more or too much thyroid in order to slow down thyroid hormone production.

If it feels like 70 degrees in a room and the thermostat is set on 70 degrees, everything is fine and dandy in your world. However, if the thermostat is set on 70 degrees, yet there is ice on the windows and you can see your breath, it would be a safe assumption that something is wrong with the thermostat and it is not accurately measuring the temperature of the room.

So if you have all the symptoms of hypothyroidism, yet your blood tests are normal, there's a good chance that there may be something wrong with your pituitary gland. You don't have to wear a white coat to understand this; it's common sense.

HORMONES DECLINE AS YOU AGE

As you and I age, our risk for becoming overweight or obese and developing high blood pressure, diabetes, heart disease, cancer, osteoporosis, degenerative arthritis, and Alzheimer's disease increases. Were you worried about these diseases in your twenties? Something is happening to your body as you age that increases your susceptibility to disease. It is caused by the gradual and steady decline in the production and utilization of your naturally occurring hormones. As you age, your glands produce less and less hormones, the chemical messengers that instruct your cells what to do. This applies to all of your hormones: sex hormones, adrenal hormones, and thyroid hormones. In Great Britain and the United States, the incidence of hypothyroidism rises abruptly after menopause in women and after the age of 60 in men.[18] Accordingly, it is documented that 10–15 percent of postmenopausal women have mild, low-grade hypothyroidism, whereas in men the prevalence is 6 percent. These results are based only on blood tests. The actual incidence of hypothyroidism in both groups is significantly higher but is overlooked by many doctors.

Not only is the decline in thyroid hormone part of aging, but there are also additional factors that contribute to its diminishment:

- An infection can temporarily lower thyroid levels.
- An earlier treatment of an overactive thyroid, called hyperthyroidism, can cause lowered thyroid hormones.
- Some medications, such as corticosteroids and beta-blocker blood pressure medications, adversely affect the cells' ability to use thyroid hormones.
- Fluoride in the water, toothpaste, food products, and household items can adversely affect the ability to produce and use thyroid hormones.
- Chemicals in the environment can affect your ability to make and use thyroid hormones.
- Sex hormone decline and imbalance unfavorably affect thyroid function.
- Autoimmune disease is detrimental to thyroid hormone production.

FAULTY STANDARDS

It is important to note that the lab ranges that we mentioned earlier are often adjusted for age. What that means is that we are benchmarking with others in our age group who have low hormone levels as well. But your hormone level should be compared to the hormone levels of those who are in the prime of their life and who are feeling well. If you are 40, 50, or 60, do you want hormone levels that are average for 40, 50, or 60-year-old people, or do you want your hormone levels to be where they were during the prime of your life?

Frequently, my guests have informed me that their physicians have told them that their thyroid hormone levels were at the low end of the range but did not require treatment. This doesn't make sense. Let's say that you are driving from Houston to Dallas. When you pull into a gas station before you start on your journey, you have only 1/16 of a tank of gas left. What if the filling station attendant, when he comes to your car, says, "Sir, I'm sorry but you still have 1/16 of a tank of gas left." You would probably reply, "But I need a full tank to get to Dallas." "Sorry," the attendant replies, "but you can't fill up your gas tank until you are completely empty." Sound ridiculous? I agree. I want my car's gasoline tank full when I go on a trip. In the same way, I want my hormones at optimal levels every day. I don't want to wait until my hormones are sputtering along on empty.

TARA'S STORY

Tara grew up in a small town in Texas prior to graduating from the University of Texas at Tyler. She was an active and healthy girl, involved in cheerleading and sports through high school and college. However, during her early twenties, she began to experience frequent bouts of sinus infections, which she attributed to allergies. She took multiple rounds of antibiotics for the recurrent infections. At the age of 24, her doctor removed her tonsils in an attempt to address the frequent sore throats and sinus infections. Her throat improved, but the sinus infections were not alleviated at all. Tara said, "I was on allergy medicine pretty much throughout the year. I lived on Sudafed. I had lots and lots of allergy problems. I tried all the allergy medications, the Zyrtec, the Allegra." In spite of this, though she didn't feel great, she didn't feel it was that big a deal.

THE PREGNANCY THAT CHANGED EVERYTHING

A year after marrying her husband, Tara got pregnant with her first child. It was a difficult pregnancy. Tara felt sluggish, tired, and achy most of the time. Even though she had extremely high blood pressure with more than two months left in her pregnancy, Tara was allowed to travel from Oklahoma, where she lived at the time, to Texas for Christmas with her family. While there, on Christmas Eve, ten weeks prior to her due date, she went into labor and delivered her daughter prematurely. Tara explained, "I never figured out why I had her early, but I did have a doctor later say his guess would be a thyroid issue. After I gave birth to her, my whole existence spiraled out of control."

If you have had the joy of bringing a newborn into the world, you know that it can be the most exhilarating, yet the most exhausting, of all life experiences. Now imagine that your newborn has to spend her first four weeks in the neonatal intensive care unit. The stress on new parents can be excruciating. Tara handled it well for the first four weeks, but then her debilitating headaches began. She questioned the obstetrician about the likelihood that the headaches were related to the hormonal changes of the postpartum period. He told her, "No, that is impossible. Hormones don't cause headaches." Tara self-medicated with, in her words, "tons of Advil." Over the next several months, Tara dealt with the demands of a colicky baby who never slept through the night. About that time, during her follow up with her ob/gyn, she was asked, "Are you enjoying being a mom?" Tara's answer at the time was, "No." She explained, "Now that I look back, I think to myself, does anybody really enjoy the first one—a preemie—you know, the worst-case scenario all the way around? Who says 'yes'? You're lying if you say 'yes.'"

Her ob/gyn immediately pulled out her prescription tablet and said, "Oh my goodness, well, we need to get you on some antidepressants," and prescribed Zoloft. Tara felt hopeful and excited. She left thinking, "I'm going to feel like a new woman!" Unfortunately, reality turned out to be completely the opposite.

DESCENT INTO DARKNESS

"After I'd been taking the Zoloft for two weeks, I wanted to kill myself," Tara said. "I never had any thoughts of injuring my baby girl. I just, for whatever reason, could completely rationalize me not being here anymore. I could talk to anybody about it, just like I'm talking to you. I would just tell my husband, 'You know, I just don't want to *be* here anymore.' He didn't really know that I meant it like, on earth."

Tara eventually figured out how she was going to make that happen and mentioned it to her husband. "I thought, 'I'm just going to wrap all this up.' He was, like, 'Whoa! Wait a minute! That's crazy!'" By then it was March. The baby had been born in December. "My husband loaded me in the car that day and took me to my ob/gyn," Tara said. "We told her everything." The prescription: an appointment with a psychiatrist—in November, another eight months away.

Tara's husband said, "This is crazy! She wants to kill herself." He was instructed to take her to an emergency room, but Tara refused. Tara could hear her mom saying, "You have *never* thought these thoughts. Never!" She could hear her husband saying, "This is totally not your personality." She could hear their reasoning and think, "That's right. That's true." After discussing it further, Tara and her husband came to the agreement that Tara would stop taking the medication immediately. However, the next day, they went to see her family doctor. He said, "Well, we just need to change your antidepressant."

LITTLE IMPROVEMENT

He prescribed Effexor, which Tara stated, "was probably the worst thing to ever happen to me. It was horrible."

The side effects from the drug were severe. And, while she no longer had thoughts of suicide, she lost all maternal feelings for her baby. She felt exhausted.

"We had to call friends to come and take care of her because I couldn't even take care of her or myself. I was in bed—literally couldn't get out of bed. When I look back, it's just a sad thing. It literally went on for just months."

"I had been to two family doctors and my ob/gyn. After starting the Zoloft and the Effexor, I just kept gaining weight, gaining weight, gaining weight. By March, after the baby was born, I'd lost all of my pregnancy weight. But, as of August, I had gained 50 pounds and now weighed 180. My mom kept saying, 'That's got to be from the medicine you take.' Every doctor I would go to, I would ask about it. But they all said, 'No, that's crazy.'"

Tara had taken a semester off to care for her baby. She was hoping that once school started, she would get back into the swing of things. When the time came to return, she said, "At that point, though, honestly, I was scared, just lost. I made the decision to just not take the antidepressants anymore."

DROPPING THE MEDS

Tara stopped her medications. As a result, she was physically ill for two weeks, enduring shaking, sweating, vomiting, and insomnia.

She suffered from something her physician called "brain tremors." Those symptoms were the side effects of withdrawing from the antidepressant.[19]

"One day, I happened to mention it to my chiropractor. He told me to do a saliva test to find out what was wrong. The saliva test showed that I had adrenal fatigue. They put me on some vitamins to help, which really was the first thing that ever helped at all, but it was still so far from fixing the problem. It just made life livable. At that point, I just came to terms with the fact that I was tired and overweight. My marriage began to suffer because I wasn't who I used to be, physically or mentally. It was hard. I wasn't the mom I wanted to be. I wasn't the daughter I wanted to be. I wasn't the teacher I wanted to be."

Tara had also had a molar pregnancy during that period of time and was eventually evaluated by an endocrinologist who diagnosed her with Hashimoto's thyroiditis, also known as autoimmune thyroiditis. This is an immune system dysfunction in which the immune system attacks the thyroid gland. He prescribed Synthroid for her. But it produced no alleviation of her symptoms at all.

TURNING A CORNER

Tara first came to the Hotze Health & Wellness Center after she and her husband moved back to Texas from Oklahoma to be closer to an ill family member. We evaluated and treated her for hypothyroidism, hormonal imbalances, and nutritional deficiencies. Her tank needed to be refueled, not with drugs, but with the same molecules that God had placed in her body in the beginning. She gradually phased in different parts of our treatment program, starting with a much-needed boost for her adrenal fatigue with bioidentical cortisol. She said that for the first time *in her life* she slept through the night.

Not only that, she felt rested. And this occurred just a few days after first visiting our center! She implemented a yeast-free eating program designed to detoxify her body and support it nutritionally. Synthroid was replaced with desiccated thyroid, which is biologically identical to that made by our bodies.

Tara told me that within ten days she felt like a completely new person. She said that over the next eight months, in addition to enjoying the return of her health and energy, she lost 56 pounds, even though she didn't routinely exercise. No more headaches, allergy symptoms, extra weight, or depressed moods.

In spite of the hellish four years that Tara had spent in a progressively downward spiral, she is one of the lucky ones. Because many of the symptoms of low thyroid, such as the fatigue and depressed moods that Tara experienced after giving birth, are usually addressed by mainstream doctors with antidepressants and other drugs, I am certain that millions of individuals just like Tara are suffering in the same way.

SUMMARY

1. Hypothyroidism is diagnosed by measuring your basal body temperature and evaluating your clinical symptoms.
2. Thyroid hormones affect every cell and organ in your body.
3. People don't lie, but lab tests do.
4. Hormones decline as we age and need to be replenished for our bodies to function optimally.
5. For more information, please visit www.hotzehwc.com/PatientsDontLie.

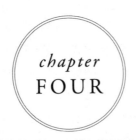

chapter
FOUR

HOW DOES HYPOTHYROIDISM OCCUR?

CASSIE'S STORY

"I think I had always struggled with my weight, but I could always keep it under control. And then I had my first child."

Cassie had never been the "thin girl." In fact, she had struggled with her weight since her teenage years, in spite of leading a very active lifestyle. She played competitive sports through high school and was an avid runner in college. Even though she ran every day and maintained disciplined eating habits, it was always a battle. It was a battle she won, until she had her first child.

Cassie, a psychologist, minister's wife, and young mother, described to me her frustration and sense of helplessness over the next couple of years. Cheerful, determined, and motivated, she began to power through a workout schedule that included total body conditioning classes four to five times each week. At the same time, she and her husband started a new church, built its new building, grew the church membership from 500 members to 1700 members, and had a second child. She said, "It was stressful, but a good stress." Cassie nursed both of her kids, continued to exercise, and ate healthfully. Unfortunately, her body did not respond to these efforts, and as she put on the pounds, she felt defeated. As she watched her friends nurse their children, work out, and eat a balanced diet but get completely different results than she did, she began to ask, "Why?"

As if the weight gain wasn't upsetting enough, Cassie also suffered from extreme fatigue. Her first thought upon awakening in the morning was, "How long until the morning nap?" Getting up from the morning nap, she focused on making it until the afternoon nap. She grew increasingly impatient, frustrated, and irritable. One day, thinking enough was enough, she went to see her beloved ob/gyn.

COMMON EXPERIENCE

Cassie explained to her doctor her predicament. She was shaken by his proclamation. "Cassie, we have got to work on this weight because you are *obese!*" She left his office with the word rattling around and around in her thoughts. She was indignant that his advice consisted of: "You just need to eat less and exercise more." Since that had been the plan she had been following throughout the difficult period of her children's births, she knew that wasn't the answer. Cassie bawled all the way home.

As luck would have it, or through divine intervention as Cassie believes, at about that time, she was given my first book, *Hormones, Health, and Happiness*, by one of her friends, who said, "Just read this. I watch you, and I know you, and just read it." So she did. And as she read, more tears flowed, but this time she cried because she found herself described in the book. Over and over, she exclaimed to herself, "That's me! That's me!"

With her husband's full support, Cassie sought help at our center, where her doctor listened to her story and put the fragmented puzzle pieces of her medical history and symptoms together to find a solution. She came to understand that through the years her thyroid, female, and adrenal hormonal foundation had crumbled and she needed to replenish the hormones that were missing. She began taking natural desiccated thyroid, bioidentical progesterone, and vitamins, and began an eating program that focused on cleansing her body of yeast.

Her energy returned. As her doctor slowly increased her dose of natural desiccated thyroid, her symptoms and her extra pounds began to disappear. She felt enthusiastic again and lost 40 pounds within the first three months. Every once in a while, she encourages people who are dealing with the same difficulties she previously endured to read the book that changed everything for her. She laughed as she told me, "I felt like I got my life back, but my husband likes to say he got his wife back!"

WHY ME AND WHY NOW?

Now that we have shown you how to identify hypothyroidism clinically, let's talk about how and why it can occur. At this point, you may believe you have hypothyroidism due to your symptoms but are asking why. Like Cassie, or the other guests whose stories you have read in this book, you may have been healthy throughout your life, but then things changed for the worse, and you do not understand how this has happened. This chapter is written to provide you with an understanding of the causes of hypothyroidism.

A MULTITUDE OF FACTORS

The majority of hypothyroidism cases result from problems that start within the thyroid gland itself. Thyroid function is also affected when there are problems with either of the thyroid gland's two helpers, the pituitary gland and the hypothalamus. The thyroid function declines when environmental factors adversely affect your cells' ability to receive and use thyroid hormones.

Each of these primary concerns is complex in and of itself, and the complexity only increases the more closely we examine them. We often have to look at factors beyond the thyroid gland and its main helpers to understand hypothyroidism. Your hormone glands and the hormones they produce are intended to work together in harmony to keep you vibrant and full of energy. Thyroid hormones exist in a delicate balance with your other hormones, your gastrointestinal system, your insulin level, your diet, and with vitamins and minerals.

We'll be discussing a number of these factors in greater detail, but you may find it helpful to look at the road map before we start our journey. The major causes of hypothyroidism include:

- autoimmune thyroid disease
- sex hormone imbalance and decline; estrogen dominance in women
- hysterectomies followed by treatment with only estrogen hormones
- sex hormone decline in men
- adrenal fatigue
- aging and hormonal decline in both females and males
- fluoride poisoning of the thyroid
- iodine deficiency
- cellular resistance to thyroid hormones

- surgical removal or radioactive destruction of the thyroid gland
- some pharmaceutical drugs, especially beta blockers for high blood pressure and lithium for depression

INFLAMMATION AND AUTOIMMUNITY

You are familiar with inflammation. If you were to puncture your foot with a nail, that area of your foot would begin to swell, turn bright red, and eventually become warm to the touch. This is what you see and feel on the surface level.

What you are not able to see is that your white blood cells have released chemicals to protect you from bacteria, viruses, or other foreign substances and have increased blood flow to the affected area. This is the inflammatory response.

The inflammatory response is your body's reaction to injury, like an army sending reinforcements to a battle. Your immune system has received the call that help is needed, and it is there to protect you from further injury. In the case of acute injury, such as the nail puncture incident, the inflammatory response is essential to the body's healing process.

WHEN INFLAMMATION BECOMES CHRONIC

In disease processes, the inflammation does not subside and can cause numerous health problems. You may be familiar with words that end in "itis" that are used by physicians to describe inflammation of the tissue or organs. A few examples include arthritis, tendonitis, and hepatitis. In some diseases, the body's immune system inappropriately initiates an inflammatory response against itself when there are no invading marauders to fight. In these cases, your immune system begins to attack its own tissues, responding as if normal organs or tissues are the problem. This is called an autoimmune disease.

Two different autoimmune diseases involve the thyroid, Graves Disease (too much thyroid hormone), and Hashimoto's Disease (too little thyroid hormone). Since our focus is on hypothyroidism, let's take a closer look at Hashimoto's disease caused by autoimmune thyroiditis.

ATTACK OF THE "ITISES"

These are some of the more common maladies ending in "itis" that involve inflammation of particular body parts, as noted:

- arthritis = joint
- hepatitis = liver
- myocarditis = heart muscle
- thyroiditis = thyroid gland
- bursitis = bursa (fluid-filled sacs that cushion bones and tendons)
- tendonitis = tendon

AUTOIMMUNE THYROIDITIS
(HASHIMOTO'S DISEASE)

Autoimmune thyroiditis is a disease state of the immune system that leads to hypothyroidism. It is also known as Hashimoto's disease, having been named after Dr. Hakaru Hashimoto, a Japanese physician, who first described it in 1912, while working in Germany.

With autoimmune thyroiditis, an individual's immune system produces antibodies that attack the thyroid gland, causing inflammation and glandular damage, resulting in a decreased ability to produce adequate amounts of thyroid hormone. Antibodies also bind to the circulating thyroid hormones in the blood, making them less available to the cells. Unfortunately, most physicians do not routinely perform blood tests to determine if their patients have autoimmune thyroiditis, which, if present, might explain the reason for their hypothyroid symptoms. It is extremely common for patients who have autoimmune thyroiditis to otherwise have normal routine thyroid blood tests. Routine thyroid blood tests do not reveal the presence of autoimmune thyroiditis, which affects the cells' ability to utilize thyroid hormones. This is one of the reasons that hypothyroidism often remains undiagnosed.

If you have symptoms of hypothyroidism, your blood should be specifically tested to determine if you have autoimmune thyroiditis. This can be done by having your blood checked for two thyroid antibodies:

1. Thyroid peroxidase antibodies (TPOAB) and
2. Antithyroglobulin antibodies (ATA)

In his book *Why Do I Still Have Thyroid Symptoms When My Lab Tests Are Normal?* Dr. Datis Kharrazian introduced me to the relationship between gluten sensitivity and autoimmune thyroiditis.[20]

THE GLUTEN CONNECTION

What causes the immune system to make antibodies against the thyroid gland? Interestingly, it may result from what you eat, specifically grain products such as wheat, rye, and barley. In individuals with healthy intestines, grain products do not routinely cause a problem. But when an individual has inflammation of the intestines, a leaky gut syndrome may occur. In leaky gut syndrome, the lining of the intestines becomes inflamed and impaired, allowing for food proteins, such as gluten, bacterial byproducts, and other toxins, to enter the blood stream. When this occurs, the immune system reacts to these foreign proteins by making antibodies to destroy them. These antibodies may then cross-react and attack various organs and tissues in the body. This is the likely cause of autoimmune disease.

There are several blood antibody tests that can determine if you are making antibodies to gluten. When the presence of gluten antibodies is associated with the gastrointestinal symptoms of bloating, gas, indigestion, diarrhea, and other diffuse symptoms, such as headaches, joint pain, fatigue, hair loss, rashes, and infertility, among others, a gastrointestinal specialist will usually recommend a biopsy of the upper small intestine, the duodenum. If there are specific pathologic changes, a diagnosis of celiac disease is made. Celiac disease is inflammation of the lining of the bowels, as described above, leading to leaky gut syndrome. But did the gluten cause the inflammatory changes in the bowel lining or was it something else? The only treatment is a gluten-free diet. This means the elimination of all grain products, specifically wheat, barley, and rye.

OTHER FACTORS IN THE GUT

It may be that the intestinal inflammation was caused by something other than gluten, such as yeast overgrowth caused by antibiotic use, bacterial or viral infections, or by chemicals and toxins in your diet. Once you have leaky gut syndrome, food proteins and other foreign substances cross the defensive lining of the intestines.

The immune system will inevitably attack these food proteins, leading to food allergies. This then causes further inflammation of the bowel lining and worsening of the leaky gut syndrome.

Blood tests can be performed to determine if you are allergic to any foods. But what caused the inflammation of the bowels and leaky gut syndrome in the first place?

In most cases, the cause of leaky gut syndrome is due to antibiotic use, which destroys normal, beneficial bacteria in the large intestine, allowing for yeast overgrowth.

There is a healthy balance between the beneficial bacteria in the gut and yeast, which is a type of fungus known as candida albicans. When antibiotics are taken, this balance is disrupted. When yeast overgrows, it destroys the lining of the small intestine that functions as a protective barrier, allowing food proteins, bacterial byproducts, other toxins, and chemicals to pass through the lining and into the blood stream.

THE CYCLE OF ILLNESS

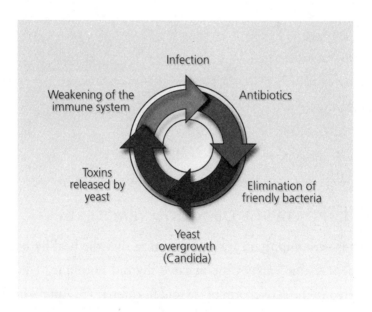

The immune system's reaction to these foods and other undigested products stimulates an inflammatory response every time they enter the bloodstream. This compounds the leaky gut syndrome. As discussed previously, the immune system reacts by producing antibodies to these toxic substances. As these foods and other products circulate in the blood, they must then be detoxified by the liver and excreted into the bile. When the liver's ability to detoxify these products is compromised, they remain in the bloodstream and are deposited in the various tissues of the body instead. Now the individual has not only a stressed immune system, but also a toxic load in the tissues. Inevitably, there is a spiraling down into poor health and disease.

COMMON FOOD ALLERGIES

It's possible to develop an allergy to any food, but some are implicated much more than others. Some of the most likely culprits include:

- wheat
- corn
- egg
- milk
- yeast
- soybean
- coconut

THE IMPORTANCE OF "GOOD" BACTERIA

It is very important for you to realize that the healthy bacteria in your intestine enables the inactive thyroid hormone, T4, to be converted to the active form of thyroid hormone, T3. Approximately 20 percent of this conversion takes place in the intestines. When some of the healthy bacteria are destroyed by antibiotics, an imbalance occurs in the normal bacterial makeup of the intestine. This prevents the proper conversion of T4 to T3. It is one of the reasons that you can have normal T4 levels in your blood but not have adequate levels of T3 in your cells.

If this has occurred with you, it is essential that you clean up your eating habits and start on a yeast-free eating program, eliminating sugar and all simple carbohydrates, including bread, potatoes, rice, and desserts. You should also eliminate any food products to which you have been found to be allergic. There are some pharmaceutical medications that may be required to kill the yeast as well. Ultimately, you must adopt a healthy eating program.

Hippocrates, the father of medicine, who lived from 460 to 370 BC, wrote, "Let food be your medicine and let medicine be your food." These words of wisdom remain true today.

> *"Let food be your medicine and let medicine be your food."*
> **—HIPPOCRATES**

AUTOIMMUNE THYROIDITIS AFTER PREGNANCY

In women, autoimmune thyroiditis often occurs during or after pregnancy leading to postpartum hypothyroidism. This may be caused by the imbalance between the estrogen and progesterone hormones that occurs after delivery when progesterone levels plummet. This leads to estrogen dominance, which dysregulates the immune system.

Autoimmune thyroiditis often goes undiagnosed after pregnancy because the physician only orders routine thyroid tests and does not check for antibodies to the thyroid gland. When the routine thyroid blood tests return within the "normal" range, the new mother's symptoms are often attributed to postpartum depression, and she is prescribed antidepressants. This is tragic because antidepressants never resolve the problems caused by hypothyroidism, but they can cause a host of adverse side effects of their own. In this case, all the mother needs is desiccated thyroid USP and some bioidentical progesterone to restore her hormonal balance and get her feeling well again.

SEX HORMONE DECLINE IN WOMEN

Why do more women suffer from hypothyroidism than men? Genetically, women are more likely to inherit autoimmune thyroiditis, which is one of the reasons why women are affected by hypothyroidism six times more frequently than men. The studies conducted at the Hotze Health & Wellness Center have demonstrated that 32 percent of the women and 18 percent of the men evaluated at the center had autoimmune thyroiditis. This is a much higher incidence than in the general population where 10 percent of adults have detectable thyroid antibodies. Genetics aside, there is one more factor behind the higher incidence of hypothyroidism found in women, that being hormone imbalance.

Hormonal changes mark the seasons in a woman's life. Her hormones will fluctuate over the years: at the onset of her menstrual cycles, known as puberty; and during her monthly menstrual cycles, pregnancies and births, perimenopause, and menopause. Her hormones may become imbalanced at any of these crossroads.

THE DANCE OF HORMONAL BALANCE

How do hormones function and influence women's moods, feelings, and energy levels? Moreover, how does hormonal imbalance contribute to hypothyroidism?

- Estrogen is primarily a female hormone that is produced by the ovaries and stimulates cell division and promotes the proliferation of cells, particularly the inner lining of the womb (uterus). Estrogen is produced beginning on day one of the menstrual cycle and the levels vary throughout the menstrual cycle.

- Progesterone is produced by the ovaries after ovulation occurs, between days 15 and 28 in a normal menstrual cycle. Progesterone balances the effect of the estrogen hormone by maturing the inner lining of the womb, preparing it to receive new life. Progesterone promotes gestation, hence its name. It plays a protective role during pregnancy. During a normal menstrual cycle, estrogen dominates the first half of the cycle until ovulation, and progesterone dominates the second half until menstruation. Together, both hormones orchestrate this harmonious female monthly dance.

Progesterone is essential to thyroid hormone production; it stimulates the enzyme thyroperoxidase in the thyroid gland, which causes the production of thyroid hormones, T3 and T4, from the protein thyroglobulin. Progesterone also appears to enhance the thyroid receptors in the cells, making it easier for thyroid hormones to be assimilated.

Progesterone is also an important brain hormone in both men and women.[21]

Unfortunately, as the ovaries age, progesterone and estrogen can fall out of balance, resulting in a condition called estrogen dominance.

--------- **WORD WISE** ---------

Estrogen. We tend to think of estrogen as a single hormone, but it's actually a class of hormones consisting of three separate and distinct molecules: estriol, estradiol, and estrone.

ESTROGEN DOMINANCE

Although a woman's menstrual cycle is a balancing act between estrogen and progesterone, estrogen has developed a bad reputation over the years. There are many reasons for this, which will be covered in more depth in a later chapter. However, what I have found in the treatment of tens of thousands of women is that estrogen is not dangerous as long as it is given in normal physiological doses in balance with progesterone. Estrogen dominance occurs when it is not in balance with progesterone.[22] This is also correctly referred to as progesterone deficiency.

A number of factors can cause estrogen to dominate in the body, including the aging process. All hormones decline as we age. However, progesterone levels fall much more rapidly than estrogen levels. By the time a woman reaches menopause, her progesterone level is likely to be 1/120 of what it was in her twenties. In comparison, estrogen levels will have declined by only 40 percent by the time a woman reaches menopause. This is largely because the ovaries are not the only source of estrogen in the body. Fat cells produce estrogen as well. For this reason, postmenopausal women who are obese will have higher levels of estrogen than thin postmenopausal women. All of these factors contribute to creating estrogen dominance.

PATHWAY TO HYPOTHYROIDISM

You may be wondering what all of this has to do with hypothyroidism.

Estrogen dominance also causes the liver to produce increasing levels of a protein called thyroid-binding globulin (TBG). TBG does just what its name suggests: it binds thyroid hormone in the blood, preventing it from being used by the cells of your body.

Imagine that you are walking up to your front door and just before you reach into your pocket to get your keys, someone jumps you and ties your hands behind your back and binds your feet. Now, what are your chances of unlocking the door with the key? When TBG encounters free thyroid hormone in your blood, it latches on to that thyroid hormone, making it no longer free and available to enter your cells and to regulate your metabolism. You may have adequate thyroid hormone levels in your blood, but they cannot be adequately assimilated by your cells. This results in hypothyroidism. Every woman will inevitably develop estrogen dominance and experience the symptoms and develop the signs of hypothyroidism, to one degree or another, as she marches through her menstrual life.

Women's problems are further compounded by the fact that birth control pills and postmenopausal estrogen supplementation unbalanced by progesterone exacerbates estrogen dominance, leading to increasing levels of TBG and hypothyroid symptoms.

In contrast, the male hormone testosterone has no effect on TBG, and actually stimulates the conversion of the inactive thyroid hormone, T4, to the active thyroid hormone, T3, within the cells. It's no mystery, then, why women are much more likely than men to experience hypothyroidism.

HYSTERECTOMY

During my surgical internship, I became familiar with the surgeon's motto, "a chance to cut is a chance to cure." Too often medicine chooses to remove the affected organ rather than to search for the underlying cause of its diseased state. Hysterectomies often fall into this misguided surgical mentality. Broda Barnes, MD, was one of the first to point out that thyroid difficulty or untreated thyroid issues can lead to unnecessary hysterectomies. Barnes was a pioneer in the field of thyroid research and treatment. He found that desiccated thyroid treatment in women patients with hypothyroidism not only reduced unnecessary hysterectomies, but also controlled fibroid tumors, and eliminated ovarian cysts and excessive menstrual flow. Before we choose drastic measures, why not consider hypothyroidism and treat it appropriately?

Of course, once women undergo a hysterectomy, during which the ovaries are also removed, they are placed on hormone replacement therapy, which is usually Premarin, estrogen derived from pregnant mares' urine. Much of this mare-derived estrogen is not identical to the estrogen made by women. It is routinely given without providing progesterone to balance the estrogen. This throws women into a state of estrogen dominance.

SEX HORMONE CHANGES IN MEN

Larry's job in sales required a high level of physical and mental stamina. Yet, over a six-year period, he noticed a decline in his drive and energy. His first doctor put him on Accupril for high blood pressure, and later, he prescribed Lipitor when Larry's cholesterol was elevated. Every time another symptom appeared, the doctor had another pill. It was affecting Larry's personal life. His libido and sexual potency began to wane. Because of the latter, Larry also requested that his testosterone level be checked. The results revealed that his testosterone level was in the low range of normal for a man his age, but according to his doctor, "not low enough to treat." However, his doctor did have a drug for his erectile dysfunction: Viagra.

Let me make this crucial point. No man has erectile dysfunction or impotency because he has low levels of Viagra in his body. When men are entering puberty, their mothers don't wake them up in the morning and say, "Here son, take your Viagra today so that you can be a man." Young men don't need Viagra. Why? Their bodies are being flooded with high levels of testosterone. The primary cause of impotency in men as they age is the inevitable decline in testosterone. Your testosterone level should not be in the "normal range" for a man your age. Rather, it should be in the range of a man in his prime at age 20.

THYROID CONVERTER

Testosterone is essential to converting the inactive thyroid hormone, T4, to the active thyroid hormone, T3. As testosterone levels decline, so do men's metabolism and energy level, and they begin to experience the symptoms of hypothyroidism. As their testosterone levels decline, they also experience a decline in their initiative, assertiveness, sense of well-being, self-confidence, goal orientation, drive, directedness, decisiveness, and analytical ability.[23] These are all brain functions. They also lose muscle mass and tone. Of course, their libido wanes, as does their potency.

Because of the positive results that Larry's wife had experienced as a patient at the Hotze Health & Wellness Center, Larry finally made an appointment for himself. Larry's hormones were replenished using desiccated thyroid USP and testosterone. He began to eat a healthy diet and take vitamin and mineral supplementation. After a year on the wellness program, Larry's cholesterol and triglycerides returned to normal. He lost 30 pounds and the inner tube around his waist disappeared. More importantly, Larry regained his drive, his mental sharpness, his energy, and physical stamina. He had eliminated all of the pharmaceutical drugs that he had been prescribed. Larry was living large and feeling like a million bucks.

MALE MENOPAUSE

Just like women, men experience a decline in their hormones as they mature. This gradual decrease in testosterone is referred to as male menopause or andropause. Men also experience a "change of life"—and their wives can probably attest to it.

Many men find they have developed that inner tube around their middle, their initiative and drive have decreased, and their stamina in the gym and bedroom isn't what it used to be. This phase in a man's life is why the phrase "grumpy old man syndrome" was coined. Men's testosterone levels slowly decline throughout midlife. By the time a man reaches the age of 50, his testosterone level is one-half to one-third of what it was in his twenties. This adversely affects his ability to utilize thyroid hormone, leading to a decrease in his metabolism. This usually produces weight gain that may be followed by high blood pressure, diabetes, heart disease, degenerative arthritis, or cancer.

Men in midlife benefit from hormone replenishment in exactly the same way women do.[24] Thyroid hormone, not to mention testosterone and cortisol, can restore a man's energy, his vitality, and his enthusiasm for life.

TEST YOURSELF ONLINE

For an online assessment of how your body and its functions are changing, test yourself on the Hotze Health & Wellness website at http://www.hotzehwc.com/Test-Your-Health/Test-Your-Health-Man.aspx.

AGING AND MIDLIFE HORMONAL CHANGES

The risk for hypothyroidism inevitably increases as we age. The aging process is due to the inevitable decline of our naturally occurring hormones. Your thyroid hormones decline with age, as do your adrenal and sex hormones. This decline brings predictable adverse effects upon your energy, your health, and your quality of life. In fact, the symptoms of hypothyroidism have become synonymous with the symptoms of aging.

This hormonal imbalance and decline negatively affects every organ and cell in your body. The degenerative problems created by hormonal decline include weight gain, high blood pressure, diabetes, heart disease, degenerative arthritis, cancer, and Alzheimer's disease, among others.

As we age, it's important that we replenish our body's foundational hormones through the use of natural, biologically identical hormones. Remember that hormones are the chemical messengers sent from key glands, particularly your thyroid gland, but also ovaries in females, testicles in males, and the adrenal glands. These chemical messengers literally inform your cells what to do and how to function. Every cell in the body needs to hear the hormone messages in order to properly function. That is why hormone replacement with desiccated thyroid USP and natural, bioidentical hormones is so essential.

THE ADRENAL FATIGUE CONNECTION
TO HYPOTHYROIDISM

The two adrenal glands, which derive their name from their location in the body (*ad* means "near"; *renal* means "kidney"), are key players in your body's response to stress. Situated on top of the kidneys, these pyramid-shaped organs, the size of walnuts, are actually two endocrine glands in one: an inner medulla, which orchestrates your short-term stress response, and an outer cortex, which mediates your adaptation to chronic stress.

The primary hormone of the medulla is epinephrine, also called adrenalin. This powerful, short-acting hormone is secreted in response to the four Es:

- exercise
- excitement
- embarrassment
- emergency

The flood of adrenaline that is unleashed in these situations causes a number of dramatic physical changes throughout your body. Your heart beats more rapidly and forcefully. Your pupils dilate and blood is shunted toward your skeletal muscles, heart, and brain. Glycogen in your liver is converted into glucose to be used for quick energy. You may break out into a cold sweat and begin breathing more rapidly. In short, your body is mobilized for action. This is why adrenaline is known as the "fight or flight" hormone.

Adrenaline's effects are dramatic and unmistakable, but because this hormone does not linger in your body, its effects are also relatively short-lived. On the other hand, cortisol, the stress hormone produced by the outer cortex, has more prolonged effects on your body. If adrenaline is like the whip that drives the horse faster and faster, cortisol is like the rider's boot, digging into the flank, keeping the horse going even when it's ready to quit.

The primary function of cortisol is to promote gluconeogenesis, the conversion of fats and proteins to sugar (glucose). Gluconeogenesis is an essential component of your body's adaptation to chronic stress, ensuring that your vital organs, especially your brain, heart, and skeletal muscles, have enough energy to meet the increasing workload. Additionally, cortisol assists adrenaline in stimulating the cardiovascular system, increasing the heart rate and pumping capacity and temporarily raising blood pressure.

Cortisol also decreases inflammation, which is why this hormone and its counterfeit derivatives have been used to treat inflammatory conditions, such as allergies, asthma, arthritis, and skin disorders.

Due to its metabolic effects, high levels of cortisol can be extremely damaging. People with chronically elevated levels of cortisol may have high blood sugar and insulin levels and high blood pressure; they may gain weight, especially around the abdomen, and they have a greater risk of heart disease. However, just because high levels of cortisol are harmful doesn't mean that low levels are healthy. As with all hormones, balance is the key.

A FAILURE TO ADAPT

Cortisol is essential to life. Laboratory animals that have had their adrenal glands removed can no longer produce cortisol, and they are very fragile creatures. They can function reasonably well if their environment is kept perfectly stable. However, even the slightest variation in their environment—a drop in room temperature, for example—can spell death for these creatures. With the loss of their adrenal glands, they have lost their ability to adapt.

Human beings are not laboratory animals, and the environments we live in are seldom stable. We are exposed to a constant onslaught of stressors: finances, noise, pollution, traffic, inclement weather, injuries, illnesses, emotional conflicts, deadlines, loss of loved ones, and on and on. We may heap stress on top of stress by smoking, eating refined carbohydrates, drinking coffee, or going without adequate sleep. Chronic, unrelenting stress, whether physical or psychological or both, eventually leads to adrenal fatigue.

The adrenals simply cannot produce enough cortisol to meet the demands. The result? We feel "stressed out"—because we are.

As you might expect, some of the effects of suboptimal cortisol levels are the opposite of those seen with high cortisol levels. Instead of hyperglycemia, or elevated blood sugar, individuals with mild adrenal fatigue often have hypoglycemia, or low blood sugar. Instead of high blood pressure, they may have low blood pressure. Instead of feeling mentally stimulated, they may have trouble concentrating. But the number-one symptom of adrenal insufficiency is fatigue. Whereas individuals with optimal cortisol levels have energy to burn, those with low cortisol levels drag themselves through the day, feeling exhausted.

If you have adrenal fatigue, you may function reasonably well when your life is stable but fall apart if stress is added. You are likely to be more vulnerable to infections and to heal more slowly than those with healthy adrenal glands. You may suffer from headaches, heart palpitations, or joint and muscle pain. You may develop allergies or chemical sensitivities or experience a worsening of existing allergies or asthma.

SYMPTOMS AND SIGNS OF ADRENAL FATIGUE

If the symptoms listed below look similar to those of hypothyroidism, you're right. Although they are clinically distinct conditions, adrenal insufficiency and hypothyroidism are both metabolic problems that result in a slowdown of the body's functions and a decline in energy. Some people have only one of these conditions, but many have both. If your hypothyroidism is complicated by adrenal insufficiency, it's important to address this underlying problem at the same time. The signs of adrenal failure are:

- chronic fatigue
- low blood sugar (hypoglycemia)
- low blood pressure (hypotension)
- dizziness or lightheadedness upon standing
- muscle and/or joint pain
- recurrent infections
- allergies and/or asthma
- irregular menstrual cycles
- infertility
- low libido
- headaches
- hair loss
- dry skin
- anxiety or panic attacks
- depression
- heart palpitations
- difficulty "bouncing back" from stress
- cold and heat intolerance

ADRENAL AND THYROID: PARTNERS IN HEALTH

Some patients with hypothyroidism do not regain their energy even when they are taking natural desiccated thyroid. I was puzzled by this phenomenon until I learned about Dr. Barnes' use of natural cortisol and read Dr. William McK. Jefferies' book, *Safe Uses of Cortisol*.[25] Dr. Jefferies found that adrenal fatigue often occurs in conjunction with hypothyroidism, and that, in the absence of adequate cortisol, thyroid hormone replacement was less effective.

The reason for this is that when the adrenal glands are weak, even normal thyroid activity is a burden. Adding supplemental thyroid hormone may result in initial improvement in energy levels and other symptoms, but as the adrenal glands become more exhausted, energy production is shut down. The solution is not more thyroid hormone. What is called for is adrenal support with small doses of cortisol.

In my experience, as well as that of Drs. Jefferies and Barnes, low-dose cortisol can make a tremendous difference in the energy and well-being of patients with hypothyroidism. Not only does it improve energy, raise body temperature, and increase resistance to infection, it also helps the body utilize thyroid hormone.[26]

Natural cortisol is especially helpful for patients with autoimmune thyroiditis[27], the common cause of hypothyroidism that I discussed earlier. Like other autoimmune conditions, autoimmune thyroiditis can develop when the adrenal glands are stressed, especially following pregnancy or at menopause.

As documented in Dr. Jefferies' book, natural cortisol actually reduces levels of thyroid antibodies, enhancing the effectiveness of thyroid hormone.

FLUORIDE POISONING OF THE THYROID:
DR. BARRY DURRANT-PEATFIELD

The English physician, Dr. Barry Durrant-Peatfield, has written extensively on hypothyroidism and its relationship to fluoride in our water supply. It is his writings that caused me to ask the following question. Could fluoride in the water supply of most cities be an unrecognized cause of hypothyroidism in the United States today?

On the periodic table of the 118 chemical elements that exist in nature, fluorine is listed in the class of halogens, which include chlorine, bromine, and iodine. Fluoride is the negative ion of fluorine. When introduced into the human body, fluoride acts as a poison in your system and inhibits the activity of enzymes necessary for the production of thyroid hormones. Enzymes are specialized proteins that stimulate biochemical reactions within our cells.

Fluoride may be found in tap water, toothpaste, nonorganic foods, pesticides used in farming, dental products, some chewing gum, many household cleaning products, and numerous other commonly used products. You come in contact with it daily, especially if your city's water supply has been fluoridated. As of 2012, nearly 70 percent of Americans drink fluoridated water.

Fluoridated tap water was a public health measure initiated by city governments in 1945, with the goal of decreasing dental cavities in children. Studies in several cities, during the late 1940s and early 1950s, appeared to show a decline in cavities in children who drank fluoridated water. These studies, which have since been discredited, led to numerous cities adopting the policy of fluoridating their water supply. Studies indicate that there is no difference in the incidence of tooth decay between the United States and Western Europe, which does not fluoridate its water.

Yet, given official warnings about fluoride, it hardly seems like a substance you should be ingesting. Fluoride is a toxic byproduct of the aluminum and fertilizer industries. What these industries would normally have to dispose of as a toxic waste is now sold to American cities to fluoridate their water. Studies indicate that fluoride is a neurotoxin that decreases the IQ of children. Not only is it a poison, but 50 percent of what you ingest accumulates in your body.

OFFICIAL WARNINGS ABOUT FLUORIDE

- The Material Safety Data Sheet (MSDS), which is required by the federal government for all hazardous products, lists the following warning about chronic exposure to fluoride:

   Chronic Exposure to Fluoride: Chronic inhalation and ingestion may cause chronic fluoride poisoning (fluorosis) characterized by weight loss, weakness, anemia, brittle bones, and stiff joints. Effects may be delayed. Chronic exposure may cause lung damage. Laboratory experiments have resulted in mutagenic effects. Chronic exposure to fluoride compounds may cause systemic toxicity. Skeletal effects may include bone brittleness, joint stiffness, teeth discoloration, tendon calcification, and osteosclerosis. Animal studies have reported the development of tumors.

- A more familiar warning may be the one you can find on the back of your fluoridated toothpaste. The wording goes like this: "If more than used for brushing is accidently swallowed, get medical help or contact a poison control center right away."

FLUORIDE TO REIGN IN OVERACTIVE THYROID

In the 1930s fluoride was used in a product called fluorotyrosine (trade name Pardinon), manufactured by a German pharmaceutical company named Bayer. Flourotyrosine was used to treat hyperthyroidism, which is an overactive thyroid. It poisoned the enzymes in the thyroid gland and slowed down the production of thyroid hormones. Unfortunately, some patients' thyroid glands were so poisoned by flourotyrosine that their glands were destroyed. Many patients suffered complete loss of thyroid function with this treatment. Consequently, the use of this drug for the treatment of hyperthyroidism was discontinued and, instead, it was used as a pesticide. Over your lifetime, you accumulate a toxic load of fluoride in your fat cells.

Why is all of this important? The abnormal changes in the protein structure, caused by fluoride exposure, damages the normal biochemical reactions in your body, which causes your immune system to produce antibodies to destroy these abnormal proteins. This can ultimately lead to an autoimmune reaction to the thyroid gland. Common forms of autoimmune thyroiditis are Hashimoto's thyroiditis, and Graves' disease, a less common disorder that causes an overactive thyroid gland. The enzyme poisoning effect of fluoride can eventually extend to your genes and damage your chromosomes. This can lead to a host of adverse health problems from abnormalities in newborn babies to cancer.

FLUORIDE'S DIRECT IMPACT ON THE THYROID

While fluoride has adverse effects on the immune system and triggers autoimmune disease, including autoimmune thyroiditis, it also negatively affects the thyroid gland by:

1. Poisoning the enzymes in the thyroid gland that produce thyroid hormones;

2. Adversely affecting the thyroid hormone receptors on all the body's cells; preventing the adequate uptake of thyroid hormones;

3. Inhibiting the production of TSH from the pituitary gland;

4. Displacing iodine, which is essential for producing thyroid hormones.

EUROPE: NO FLUORIDE, FEWER PROBLEMS

It's interesting to note that 34 percent of Americans are obese compared to just 8 percent of Italians and 9 percent of the French. Why is obesity four times as prevalent in the United States? Could it have something to do with the fluoridated water that 70 percent of Americans drink? Here's a clue: Italy and France do not fluoridate their water.

There is definitely a correlation between the fluoridation of water in the United States and obesity, a classical feature of hypothyroidism. This does not necessarily prove causation, but when you understand the adverse effect that fluoride has on thyroid hormone production and function, it appears that fluoride may be the likely culprit.

Public health bureaucrats and well-intentioned individuals thought that they could reduce cavities by adding fluoride to the water. They never considered the unintended adverse consequences that this might have on your health.

HOW TO REDUCE FLUORIDE EXPOSURE

What can you do to prevent exposure to fluoride? Some simple steps can go a long way:

- Make sure that you have a filtration system that removes fluoride from your drinking water.
- Use nonfluoridated toothpaste.
- Check the labels on processed food and on home cleaning products.
- Take oral iodine, which displaces fluoride and allows it to be discharged from your body. Iodoral is a product that contains iodine and potassium iodide.

IODINE DEFICIENCY

Hypothyroidism can result from iodine deficiency. The thyroid gland requires most of the iodine ingested by our body in order to make thyroid hormones. The thyroid hormones are critical to the functioning of all the other endocrine glands that produce hormones. In his book, *Iodine, Why You Need It, Why You Can't Live Without It,* Dr. David Brownstein discusses how essential iodine is for normal thyroid function, as well as how necessary it is for a healthy immune system because it contains antiviral, anticancer, and antibacterial properties.[28] Iodine deficiency exists at epidemic levels around the world.

Dr. Brownstein describes that he was taking Armour Thyroid for a diagnosed problem of hypothyroidism. When he tested himself for iodine levels with the iodine loading test, he discovered his iodine level was very low. After three months of iodine supplementation, his levels returned to normal, and he experienced a concomitant rise in his energy level. Dr. Brownstein then began to study his patients and found that 90 percent of them had iodine deficiencies. He suggested treating iodine deficiencies simultaneously with the treatment for thyroid deficiencies. We have been recommending this approach to our patients at our center for numerous years with very effective outcomes.

Remember that each thyroid hormone molecule contains either three or four atoms of iodine. The thyroid hormones are named T3 and T4, respectively. If your diet contains insufficient iodine, the thyroid gland can't synthesize adequate amounts of thyroid hormones.

INDICATIONS OF LOW IODINE

Iodine-deficiency induced hypothyroidism may be character-ized by an enlarged thyroid gland or goiter. Blood tests will generally show high levels of TSH and low levels of T4, indicating that the pituitary gland is functioning normally, but the thyroid gland is failing to respond to the signal. This type of hypothyroidism is now relatively rare in the United States because of the availability and widespread use of iodine in iodized salt.

However, goiter regions still exist in many areas of the world.[29] Since iodine deficiency remains a global public health problem, and is monitored by the World Health Organization (WHO) and United Nations Children's Fund (UNICEF), a consistent update was published as recently as September 2008.[30]

The data suggests that 31.5 percent of school-age children (266 million) worldwide have insufficient iodine intake. In the general population, an astonishing two billion people have insufficient iodine intake. Iodine deficiency is a public health problem in 47 countries.

While iodine deficiency is easily tested and treated, few individuals have ever been educated about its importance to their overall health.

INHERITANCE AND TYPE 2 HYPOTHYROIDISM

Dr. Mark Starr is the author of *Hypothyroidism, Type 2, the Epidemic* in which he documents the rising epidemic of persons with hereditary low thyroid function. The descriptions below have been reprinted with his permission and distinguish type 2 hypothyroidism[31] from what he calls type 1 hypothyroidism.

TYPE 1 HYPOTHYROIDISM

"A failure of the thyroid gland to produce sufficient amounts of thyroid hormones necessary to maintain 'normal' blood levels of those hormones and 'normal' blood levels of the thyroid stimulating hormone (TSH) produced by the pituitary gland. The TSH test is the standard blood test your doctor checks when looking for hypothyroidism. Around 7 percent of Americans are currently thought by mainstream medical practitioners to suffer from type 1 hypothyroidism."

TYPE 2 HYPOTHYROIDISM

"A peripheral resistance to thyroid hormones at the cellular level is not due to a lack of adequate thyroid hormones. Normal amounts of thyroid hormones and thyroid stimulating hormone (TSH) are detected by the blood tests; therefore, blood tests do not detect type 2 hypothyroidism. Type 2 hypothyroidism is usually inherited. However, environmental toxins may also cause or exacerbate the problem. The pervasiveness of type 2 hypothyroidism has yet to be recognized by mainstream medicine but is already in epidemic proportions."

The symptoms of types 1 and 2 are the same although the causes are different. According to Starr, type 2 hypothyroidism is inherited with either parent contributing faulty genes. The disease is increasing in greater numbers in today's children, and no existing blood tests detect it.

Just like the physicians at the Hotze Health & Wellness Center, Dr. Starr suggests that hypothyroidism can be determined through extensive family medical history, the patient's medical history, the physical exam, and the body temperature. The use of lab tests to detect the presence of thyroid antibodies can also be useful.

SURGICAL REMOVAL OR RADIOACTIVE DESTRUCTION OF THE THYROID GLAND

Graves' disease is a disorder in which the thyroid gland is hyperactive, producing too much thyroid hormone, which increases the rate of your metabolism. Commonly the thyroid gland is enlarged. The increased thyroid hormones in the blood causes an increased heartbeat, muscle weakness, disturbed sleep, irritability, heat sensitivity—all symptoms of hyperthyroidism. Doctors may use the following remedies:

- radioactive iodine ablation that destroys the thyroid gland, eliminating the production of thyroid hormones
- surgical removal of the thyroid gland (thyroidectomy)
- drugs to block the production of thyroid hormone

Radioactive ablation and thyroidectomy produce a hypothyroid condition, which most doctors treat with Synthroid. For many people this leads to years of poor health and a host of drugs to treat the symptoms of hypothyroidism. This cause of hypothyroidism can easily be remedied by supplementing with natural desiccated thyroid hormone.

YEAST: ONE MORE POTENTIAL CAUSE OF HYPOTHYROIDISM

As mentioned previously, antibiotics kill the healthy bacteria in the intestinal tract along with bad bacteria. Further distress to the digestive system is caused by consumption of chlorine, fluoride, and nonsteroidal anti-inflammatory drugs (NSAIDs) such as aspirin and ibuprofen. When you combine these with a diet filled with sugar and other simple carbohydrates, it can cause an overgrowth of yeast in the intestines.

Yeast releases neurotoxic chemicals into the bloodstream that may damage the hypothalamus and alter thyroid production.[32] Yeast may also increase the risk of autoimmune thyroiditis by causing a leaky gut syndrome, which allows food molecules, bacterial byproducts, and other toxic chemicals into the bloodstream, causing an abnormal reaction by the immune system.

At our center, we have witnessed dramatic improvement in patients being treated for hypothyroidism once they have improved their eating habits. Our yeast-free eating program promotes the consumption of fresh lean meats, vegetables, fruits, and nuts for at least one month, sometimes longer. Coupled with this is the elimination of all sugar, products containing sugar, and simple carbohydrates such as bread, pizza, pasta, potatoes and rice. This period of healthful eating allows the digestive tract time to eliminate harmful yeast and the toxins they produce. Two pharmaceutical products, Nystatin and fluconazole, are prescribed to kill yeast. We also replenish the normal healthy intestinal bacteria using probiotics such as lactobacillus acidophilus.

A GROWING EPIDEMIC

Undiagnosed hypothyroidism is an epidemic in the United States. The way to correct it is simple, but there are few physicians willing to challenge the current status quo of choosing a TSH blood test over the patient's obvious hypothyroid complaints and physical signs when making a diagnosis. Even fewer are willing to treat their patients with desiccated thyroid USP.

USP stands for United States Pharmacopeial Convention. The United States Pharmacopeial Convention (USP) is a scientific nonprofit organization that sets standards for the identity, strength, quality, and purity of medicines, food ingredients, and dietary supplements manufactured, distributed, and consumed worldwide. USP's drug standards are enforceable in the United States by the Food and Drug Administration (FDA), and these standards are developed and relied upon in more than 140 countries. Desiccated thyroid USP is an FDA-approved product that is standardized because it bears the USP initials.

At the Hotze Health & Wellness Center, we are leading a wellness revolution, with a goal to make every American aware of this insidious hypothyroid condition. We want individuals to have the chance to restore their health by determining if they have hypothyroidism and then by treating it with bioidentical, desiccated thyroid USP. The cost is low and the benefits are life changing. What would it be worth to restore your health, transform your life, and change your world, naturally?

Severe myxedema, before and after treatment

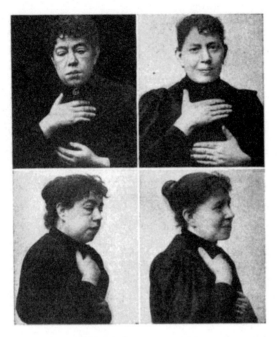

Source: Hertoghe, E. Medical Record, Sep. 1914, Vol.86, Issue 12, 489-505.

SUMMARY

1. Healthy hormone glands and the hormones they produce need to work in harmony and balance for optimal health.

2. There is a direct correlation between your cortisol levels and thyroid health.

3. Hypothyroidism can be caused by autoimmune attacks marked by chronic inflammation.

4. Factors that may trigger or exacerbate inflammation and autoimmune thyroiditis include gluten in the diet, antibiotic use, leaky gut syndrome, and yeast overgrowth.

5. Optimal thyroid health in women also depends upon a balance between estrogen and progesterone levels.

6. Both women and men have hypothyroidism, although it is six times more prevalent in women.

7. Adrenal fatigue can contribute to hypothyroidism and shares many of the same signs and symptoms.

8. Overexposure to fluoride may be a major cause of hypothyroidism in the United States.

9. For more information, please visit www.hotzehwc.com/ ThyroidHormoneConnection.

HYPOTHYROIDISM AND HEART DISEASE

I t was a crazy Saturday night in the emergency room. It must have been a full moon. I had seen everything from sore throats to snake bites and everything in between. A nurse bolted through the door into room 3 while I was examining a young man for possible appendicitis. She cried out, "Doctor, an ambulance has just pulled up with what sounds like another heart attack victim."

"Get him into the cardiac room," I said, "and I'll be right there."

There was a swirl of activity as the medics wheeled in an ashen, 50-something, balding man wearing a forest-green golf shirt, with an oxygen mask on his face. They transferred him from the gurney to the examination table. The nurses rolled in with IVs and quickly started one in each arm while another nurse hooked the patient to a cardiac monitor.

Beads of sweat covered his forehead, and he had a look of both desperation and terror. "Doctor, can you help me? It feels like something is crushing my chest."

I asked, "Do you have a history of heart problems?"

"No," he replied.

I quickly glanced at the monitor and saw that his EKG indicated the obvious. He was having a heart attack. "Give him two grams of mag sulfate IV," I ordered.

Wading into the battle, I instructed the nurse, "Let's slip some nitro under his tongue. Go ahead and give him a shot of morphine." Hopefully magnesium would regulate his abnormal cardiac rhythm and spare him from needing to be defibrillated. No sooner had I thought that then I yelled, "Get me the paddles!"

He had developed ventricular tachycardia, which required countershock therapy or else he would die. I yelled again, "Everybody stand back!"

As the paddles pressed onto his chest, I pushed the buttons on the paddles and wham! You could hear the crackle of the electricity throughout the entire room. The EKG monitor normalized for a moment and then immediately returned to its previous abnormal rhythm.

"Charge it again. Okay, stand back!"

A second time, the paddles were placed on his chest, the current discharged, and the electricity current surged through his heart. Silently, I prayed, "Dear God, please save this man's life and please help me."

Now the EKG tracing on the monitor normalized and held. I thanked God. The magnesium had taken its effect and calmed the areas of the heart that had been damaged so that they did not send off abnormal electrical pulses, which had caused the irregular heartbeats.

This occurred in the 1980s, and that is about all we had to offer a patient who was having a heart attack. If it had happened today, he would have been given intravenous drugs to thin the blood and pharmaceutical medication to control his abnormal rhythm.

The cardiologist on call had been contacted and was on his way to the hospital. The patient would stay in the emergency room until he was stable and then would be transferred to the catheterization lab where he would undergo an angioplasty in an attempt to open up his blocked coronary artery. Both his pulse and blood pressure had returned to normal and his chest pain had subsided. He was very fortunate. Had his abnormal heart rhythm developed at home before the paramedics had arrived, he would have become another sudden death statistic. Forty-seven percent of cardiac deaths occur before emergency help intervenes.

The patient's wife was standing outside the door of the cardiac room, waiting for word on her husband's condition. She was distraught. Her brows were furrowed and her eyes were moist and red. She was trembling. "Is he going to be okay?"

Encouraging her, I said, "Things are looking more hopeful than when your husband arrived. He's had a heart attack, but the cardiologist is with him now. He will be taken to the cath lab, and I feel confident that we will be able to open up his artery and take care of the problem."

She sighed with relief.

A FAMILIAR STORY

This story plays itself out again and again every day all over America. A heart attack, which is caused by blockage of the arteries of the heart, is currently the leading cause of death in America in both men and women. This year alone, approximately 750,000 Americans will die of cardiovascular disease, which includes hypertension, strokes, heart attacks secondary to coronary artery disease, atherosclerosis of other blood vessels, and diseases of the heart. Over 400,000 of these individuals will die of heart attacks caused by coronary artery disease.[33]

You probably know someone who died suddenly and without warning from a heart attack. It is the silent fear of middle-aged men—and justifiable because the first symptom of a heart problem is commonly a heart attack.

Annually, 1.2 million Americans will have a new or recurrent heart attack and six million hospitalizations occur each year due to cardiovascular disease. The annual price tag of health care, medications, and lost productivity due to cardiovascular disease has reached a total of $503.2 billion in 2010.

HYPOTHYROIDISM AND HEART ATTACKS

Ask the average person what they believe is the cause of heart attacks and you will most likely hear the following typical answers: diet, high cholesterol, high blood pressure, trans fatty acids found in margarine, heredity, or smoking. While these all may play a role in coronary heart disease, the primary and yet most unrecognized cause of heart disease is hypothyroidism.[34] If this sounds surprising, let's first get some perspective on how cardiovascular disease gained its place as modern America's top killer.

LOOKING BACK: THE AGE OF INFECTIOUS DISEASES

Since the beginning of time, man has been at war with diseases seeking to destroy his existence. The Black Plague decimated the population of Europe in the Middle Ages. Smallpox led another charge, killing children at an early age until Edward Jenner, an English physician, developed a vaccine to prevent it in 1796. Infectious diseases continued to be the leading cause of death in the Western world until the advent of antibiotics during World War II.

Of the infectious diseases, tuberculosis and pneumonia ruled the roost, cutting down large swathes of the population.

Tuberculosis attacks and destroys the lungs. It is estimated that more than one-third of the world's population is currently infected with TB, which, in its active form, kills 50 percent of victims who do not receive treatment. Ninety percent of those infected have latent infections and remain asymptomatic. Tuberculosis earned the title, Captain of Death, because it had become the leading infectious disease causing death between 1850 and 1950.

To be sure, public health measures adopted at the beginning of the twentieth century led to a reduction of tuberculosis and other infectious diseases in Western society. However, it was the discovery of penicillin by Dr. Edward Fleming and its commercialization in 1944, as well as the development of antituberculosis drugs, that knocked pneumonia, tuberculosis, and other infectious diseases from their deadly perch. In their place, coronary artery disease leading to heart attacks assumed the role as the grim reaper's new Captain of Death in the 1950s.[35]

Death patterns dramatically changed in the United States and other developed countries in the middle of the twentieth century, not as a result of changes in the environment, eating habits, or smoking, but due to the arrival of antibiotic drugs. Now people who would have died from infectious diseases, such as tuberculosis and pneumonia, were dying from heart attacks.[36]

HEART ATTACKS COME TO THE FORE

Heart attacks were an uncommon occurrence prior to 1920. Angina pectoris is the chest pain caused by restriction of coronary artery blood flow to the heart muscle and was initially described by an English physician, William Heberden in 1768.[37] Heberden was uncertain of the cause. In his textbook entitled, *Diseases of the Heart*, published in 1913, prominent Scottish cardiologist, Sir James MacKenzie, only dedicated 15 pages to the discussion of angina pectoris.[38] McKenzie attributed its cause to fatigue of the heart muscle. He does mention that in those cases in which the death of the patient with angina pectoris occurred, autopsies often revealed plaques and calcification in some of the patients' coronary arteries. There is no other discussion of coronary artery disease or of heart attacks in MacKenzie's book.

Congestive heart failure, which is a pathological condition that prevents the heart from providing circulation sufficient to allow the patient to carry out his normal daily duties, was the leading cause of death due to heart disease prior to 1950.

A SNAPSHOT OF MORTALITY

By way of capturing how the advent of antibiotics changed the nature of death in the United States, consider this: In 1900 in the United States average life expectancy was 47 years and the leading cause of death was infections. In 1950 the average life expectancy was 68 years and the leading cause of death was heart attacks due to coronary artery disease, the blockage of the arteries of the heart. Deaths from infectious diseases were in retreat.

Deaths due to heart attacks were initially categorized as caused by angina pectoris in the early part of the twentieth century. Coronary thrombosis or coronary artery disease then became popular terms used to describe the same event. There was a dramatic increase in the number of deaths caused by coronary artery disease between 1920 and 1960. Physicians and public health officials pondered this increase and came up with numerous reasons for its occurrence as mentioned earlier: diet, high cholesterol, high blood pressure, trans fatty acids found in margarine, heredity, or smoking.

AGE-OLD DISEASE

In his research of more than 70,000 autopsy reports, performed between 1930 and 1970, in Graz, Austria, Broda Barnes, MD, clearly demonstrated that coronary artery disease was not a new disease.[39] It was present in every individual whose cause of death was listed as tuberculosis, which was the leading cause of death in Europe at that time. With the advent of antibiotics these tuberculosis patients were now living long enough to die of the coronary artery disease that they already had.

In 1951 Dr. J. N. Morris reported similar findings in his review of autopsies at the London Hospital in England. While the deaths due to coronary heart disease had increased sevenfold between 1907 and 1944, the autopsy findings of damaged coronary arteries had declined slightly over the same period. It was during the first half of the nineteenth century that public health measures had been instituted. These were already reducing the incidence of infectious diseases prior to antibiotics leading to more deaths from already present and developing coronary artery disease. Dr. Morris did not recognize the relationship between infectious diseases and coronary artery disease.

In 1985 pathologist Dr. Rodney Finlayson published his review of autopsy reports between the years 1868 and 1982 at St. Bartholomew Hospital in London, England. These reports verified what Dr. Morris had discovered 24 years earlier: deaths due to coronary artery disease increased rapidly between 1910 and 1950, but the prevalence of severe coronary artery disease had remained unchanged since the turn of the century.

Dr. Barnes' exhaustive study clearly demonstrated that the rise in the death rate due to heart attacks between 1930 and 1970 was a result of the decline in the death rate due to infectious diseases that—as we saw in Chapter 2—were the scourge of people who were hypothyroid. Still, traditional medical opinion was not swayed. The usual explanation given for this increase in heart disease was too much animal fats in the diet leading to elevated cholesterol, also hypertension and smoking, among others.

INFECTION, INFLAMMATION, AND VITAMIN C

At any given life expectancy there have always been those individuals who have lived to be much older than expected and who did not contract infectious diseases or develop coronary artery disease. These individuals obviously have had a greater resistance to infections than others and do not readily develop coronary artery disease. But why? Could it be that the healthy production of thyroid hormones provides this increased resistance to infectious diseases and to the prevention of coronary heart disease?

It is well documented in the medical literature that coronary artery disease begins with an inflammatory process that damages the coronary arteries.

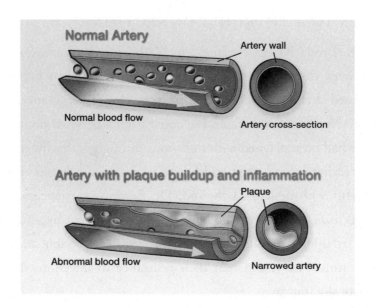

Bacteria and its antibodies have been found in the fatty deposits lining damaged coronary arteries at autopsy. It has been theorized that bacterial and viral infections cause the initial damage to the arteries, triggering the body's healing process to repair the damage. If you have adequate amounts of vitamin C and the amino acids L-lysine and proline, then collagen, the intracellular protein responsible for maintaining vascular integrity, is produced, which repairs the arterial lining. If supplies of vitamin C are inadequate, then your body is unable to make appropriate amounts of collagen to heal the arteries. Instead, it resorts to a compensatory mechanism of healing in which it uses various fat products in the blood, lipoprotein a (LPA), to patch or bandage the injury to the artery.[40]

Dr. Linus Pauling and Dr. Matthias Rath conducted experiments on guinea pigs that indicated that coronary artery disease may simply be caused by a vitamin C deficiency.[41]

CLUES TO A THYROID CONNECTION

Dr. Broda Barnes explained in his book, *Hypothyroidism: The Unexpected Illness*, the dramatic effect that the supplementation of desiccated thyroid hormones had in increasing the resistance of his patients to infectious diseases. He noted from a personal perspective that he had been plagued with infections throughout his life until he finally realized that he too had hypothyroidism and began effective treatment with desiccated thyroid. Dr. Barnes' experience was the same as mine and others who have treated patients for hypothyroidism based upon their clinical history, physical examination, and body temperature, and found that their resistance to infectious diseases dramatically improved.

The cause of coronary artery disease may be secondary to the recurrent infections that plague individuals with hypothyroidism.

In 1877 Dr. William Ord, the English physician whose pioneering work on hypothyroidism was described in the Prelude, published the autopsy findings of a 58-year-old patient of his who died with classical features of myxedema, the early term Ord coined for hypothyroidism.[42] The report described severe disease of the coronary arteries. During the same time period, surgeons in Germany were performing thyroidectomies, the removal of the thyroid gland, from patients who had severe goiters. As noted in the Prelude, within a few months, these patients would develop myxedema and die. But their autopsy reports also revealed severe coronary artery disease (CAD). From that time until the present there have been numerous case studies and medical articles describing the relationship between hypothyroidism and coronary artery disease.

Elevated blood pressure and cholesterol both have a significantly increased incidence in individuals with hypothyroidism.[43] Other risk factors for developing coronary artery disease, homocysteine and C-reactive protein (CRP), are also elevated in patients with hypothyroidism. Hypothyroidism decreases the heart's ability to contract forcefully and causes a low cardiac output state, which can lead to congestive heart failure.

Studies have demonstrated the benefit of supplemental thyroid hormones in patients who have had hypothyroidism and angina. Not only is the angina improved in more than 90 percent of the patients but the death rate is decreased.

BRODA BARNES' STUDY OF
HYPOTHYROIDISM AND HEART DISEASE

Dr. Barnes was a brilliant scientist. When a friend of his experienced a heart attack in 1950, Dr. Barnes reviewed his medical history, searching for clues. He found that his friend had suffered from symptoms of hypothyroidism for years but had not sought treatment. Could this have been a factor in his heart attack?

Dr. Barnes knew there was a relationship between hypothyroidism and high cholesterol and realized that his patients who were being treated for hypothyroidism had a remarkably low rate of heart attacks, despite the fact that the incidence of heart attacks was rising in the general population.

This observation led him to conduct a 20-year study of the relationship between supplemental desiccated thyroid hormone and reduced risk of heart attacks. He was fortunate to have a landmark study against which to compare the heart attack rate in his own patients: The Heart Disease Epidemiology study, also known as the Framingham study,[44] which began in 1949 under the sponsorship of the National Heart Institute and which continues to this day. In this study, five thousand residents of Framingham, Massachusetts, were selected to be followed medically for the rest of their lives in order to determine the cause of heart disease. Each person was followed with annual medical examinations and blood work. Their diet, smoking habits, and lifestyle were documented. However, these patients did not receive supplemental thyroid hormone.

In 1970 Dr. Barnes had 1,569 patients on natural thyroid hormone who were observed for a total of 8,824 patient years. These patients were classified by age, sex, elevated cholesterol, and high blood pressure, and compared to similar patients in the Framingham study. Based on the statistics derived in the Framingham study, 72 of Dr. Barnes' patients should have died from heart attacks. However, only four patients had done so. The heart attack death rate decreased 95 percent in patients who received natural desiccated thyroid hormone, a truly remarkable finding.

James C. Wren, MD, a Maine physician, published a similar study in the *Journal of Geriatrics Society* in 1971.[45] This five-year study was conducted on 347 patients who had documented coronary artery disease. Only 9 percent of the patients were hypothyroid by laboratory tests alone. All 347 patients were treated with desiccated thyroid hormones in physiologic doses. Cholesterol levels in this group fell by 22 percent. The mortality rate fell by 42 percent of the expected rate.

|| *The heart attack death rate decreased 95 percent in patients who received natural desiccated thyroid hormone, a truly remarkable finding.*

THE CHOLESTEROL FALLACY

Elevated cholesterol, a common feature of hypothyroidism, is considered a risk factor for developing coronary artery disease. A recent study in the *European Journal of Endocrinology*, known as the

HUNT study,[46] revealed that individuals had increasing levels of cholesterol even when the thyroid stimulating hormone (TSH) levels fell within the normal range.[47] As early as 1934, Lewis M. Hurxthal, MD, a Boston pathologist at the Lahey Clinic, recognized the relationship between hypothyroidism and elevated cholesterol levels.[48] It was so pronounced that Dr. Hurxthal considered its presence as an indication that the patient had hypothyroidism and should be treated with desiccated thyroid unless another cause could be found.

Dr. Barnes published a study in the August 1959 English medical journal, *Lancet*.[49] In the study, he treated 80 patients whose cholesterol was elevated above 200 with desiccated thyroid. In every case, cholesterol levels were reduced.

In his monograph entitled, *Thyroid Function and Its Possible Role in Vascular Degeneration*, Professor William B. Kountz demonstrated the cause and effect relationship between hypothyroidism and coronary artery disease.[50] His study demonstrated the effectiveness of using desiccated thyroid hormones, which significantly increased the life expectancy of those taking the desiccated thyroid hormone compared to a control group.

Doctors often recommend that patients with an increased risk for heart attack take a daily aspirin, cholesterol-lowering drugs such as Lipitor, and beta-blocker blood pressure medication to reduce their incidence of heart attacks. Why not consider using daily, natural, desiccated, thyroid hormone supplementation, which reduces cholesterol and decreases the death rate from heart attacks by as much as 95 percent?

CHOLESTEROL: CONSTANTLY REPLENISHED

Without cholesterol, you and I would not exist. Each cell of your body contains enzymes specifically ready to manufacture cholesterol when needed. When you were an infant, these enzymes were present in your brain, and the cholesterol levels in your central nervous system increased as you developed. As an adult, these enzymes disappear from the nervous system because the cells of the brain and spinal cord are not replaced. But aside from this exception, every other tissue in your body continues to replace cells, enabling the continuing production of cholesterol enzymes throughout your life.

CHOLESTEROL AS THREAT: THE BACK STORY

The story of how cholesterol came to play the role as the enemy of human health goes back as far as 1858. Professor Rudolph Virchow, a professor of pathology in Berlin, found that when tissue broke down, large amounts of cholesterol were released.[51] Although Virchow's results clearly showed that cholesterol was not the cause of the degradation but, rather, a byproduct, scientists began to mistakenly view cholesterol as the problem. Think of it like this. Superman was at the scene of the accident, but he wasn't the cause, he was there as part of the rescue.

The confusion was furthered 55 years later when Russian physiologist N. Anitschkow conducted an experiment in which he filled rabbits with cholesterol, resulting in changes in their arteries similar to that found in the victims of heart attacks.[52] There were numerous flaws to the study including the fact that rabbits are vegetarian and do not have the ability to metabolize cholesterol in the first place. As scientists began to replicate Anitschkow's experiments, huge amounts of cholesterol were used that would be completely unrealistic in a clinical setting. Additionally, the cholesterol that was used was not the form that humans or animals would consume and instead was either crystalline cholesterol or heat-dried egg yolk powder allowed to set for weeks. This is important because the chemical structure is changed at this point, making it an inadequate comparison to true cholesterol.

Shortly after this poorly planned study, epidemiological focus began to look at countries that consumed very low-fat—thus low-cholesterol—diets and the rate of heart attacks. On the surface, these countries looked as if they were healthier and had a lower incidence of heart disease, but as we will discuss later in this chapter, another factor was completely ignored.

Throughout the years, an amount of circumstantial evidence has been building up against cholesterol. Poorly designed studies and misinterpreted epidemiological studies have given cholesterol a bad reputation. The record has yet to be set straight by today's medicine, and today we even have institutions such as the National Cholesterol Education Program (NCEP) continuing to spread disinformation. The NCEP's purpose is to educate the American people and medical community about the dangers of high cholesterol. It is interesting to note that 88 percent of those on the NCEP board are directly paid by pharmaceutical companies.[53] These pharmaceutical companies, of course, sell cholesterol-lowering drugs. The NCEP is responsible for lowering the standard set for "normal" cholesterol levels, making a large number of Americans prime candidates for statin drugs.

FALSELY ACCUSED

Many in the medical profession, in public health, and in the pharmaceutical and food industries have hyped cholesterol as a bogey man and the cause of the increased rate of heart attacks. This is sheer nonsense! While death rates from heart attacks increased between 1920 and 1970, coronary artery disease itself has not increased over the past 130 years. This has been documented through retrospective studies of autopsy reports dating back as far as 1862. In the late nineteenth and early twentieth centuries, people did not live long enough to die of their coronary artery disease because infectious diseases killed them first.

Besides, coronary artery disease is not caused by cholesterol. It is due to inflammation caused by infections or chemicals in the environment that adversely affect the lining of the coronary arteries. Cholesterol is simply the body's compensatory healing mechanism to repair these injured arteries.

While elevated cholesterol may correlate with coronary artery disease, that does not mean that it causes it. To say that it does is a logical fallacy. A correlation is not the same as causation. As a matter of fact, autopsy results demonstrate that more than 50 percent of the individuals who died from heart attacks had normal levels of cholesterol in their blood.[54] (See Shane Ellison's book, *The Hidden Truth about Cholesterol-Lowering Drugs*.)[55]

That cholesterol could be dangerous to your health has been a marketing ploy of pharmaceutical companies and the food industry used to promote their products. Medical physicians and the public at large have swallowed this propaganda, hook, line, and sinker.

CHOLESTEROL IS VITAL TO GOOD HEALTH

If you were to ask the average person on the street, "Is cholesterol good for you or bad for you," ninety-nine percent of the time he or she would likely reply, "Bad for you!" This tells you what an effective marketing job the pharmaceutical and food companies have done. But cholesterol is essential for life[56] and 80 percent of it is manufactured in the body, primarily the liver.[57] The cholesterol in food is esterified in the digestive tract and poorly absorbed. Here are some of the important roles cholesterol plays in the body:

1. Using cholesterol as a building block, our body produces naturally occurring steroid hormones. The adrenal hormones, including pregnenolone, DHEA, and cortisol, among others, and the sex hormones, testosterone, progesterone and the estrogens, as well as vitamin D, are all derived from cholesterol. The term *steroid* was coined from the name cholesterol. Any hormone derived from cholesterol is a steroid hormone. These naturally occurring steroid hormones are necessary for good health. It is the counterfeit steroid hormones manufactured by the drug companies that are dangerous. Please take a moment to examine the cascade of hormones that are derived from cholesterol.

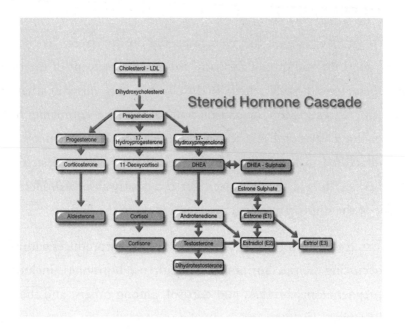

2. Your nerves depend upon cholesterol, which is required for the production of the myelin sheath that covers your nerves. Cholesterol is also essential for healthy brain function.

3. Cholesterol is a major component in the membranes that surround our cells. It gives integrity to these membranes, allowing for the proper transfer of nutrients, hormones, and waste in and out of the cells.

4. Our liver makes bile, which is stored in our gallbladders and enables us to digest fatty meals. Bile is also derived from cholesterol.

THE DANGERS OF STATIN DRUGS

Statin drugs have been the pharmaceutical companies' answer to elevated cholesterol, which I have demonstrated does not cause heart disease. Lipitor, manufactured by Pfizer, became the first drug to receive the title of mega blockbuster, bringing more than $80 billion into company coffers since its arrival on the market in 1997. Pfizer has spent nearly $258 million dollars in advertising Lipitor since 2006. "Now, I trust my heart to Lipitor" is the mantra of the actor promoting this drug during a television commercial.[58] At first, these drugs were marketed toward those with elevated cholesterol. Now they are even pushed onto healthy Americans, young and old whose cholesterol falls within the normal range. It has even been suggested that statins be given to our children. Additional statin drugs that you may recognize are Crestor, Tricor, and Zocor.

Studies have found that statin drugs lower your absolute risk for heart disease only 2 to 3 percent at best. The chance of a person benefitting from using a statin drug is two to three in 100. Further, statin drugs have only been shown to decrease heart attack and stroke by 1.4 percent and reduce the risk of death in those without risk factors by 0.3 percent. You are trading lowered cholesterol levels for memory loss,[59] muscle weakness, and pain,[60] all that goes along with hormonal imbalance, and an increased risk of cancer just for a two in 100 chance that you will benefit from a statin drug. Those don't sound like good odds to me.

You may be thinking, "If my doctor were aware of these numbers, he certainly wouldn't put me on a statin drug." Unfortunately, what your physician is seeing are the results of clinical drug trials filtered and paid for by the makers of statin drugs. Seventy-five percent of drug trials in major medical journals are funded by pharmaceutical companies. Statin drug trials are thinly veiled marketing pieces aimed at inflating the benefits of statin drugs. With a little bit of statistical magnification, drug companies are able to embellish the benefits of statin drugs and pass their health-eroding products onto unsuspecting doctors and patients.[61] You must be thinking that these are FDA-approved drugs, so surely they are safe and the benefits must outweigh the risks? But just because the FDA approves a drug does not mean that it is safe for use. Unfortunately, greed has masked the science.[62]

STATIN SIDE EFFECTS

Since cholesterol-lowering drugs have no appreciable effect on lowering your risk for heart disease, let's look at what really happens if you trust your health to statin drugs.

Statin drugs work by poisoning the enzyme acetyl-co A reductase, which is needed to produce cholesterol in the body. Every drug always has some unintended and harmful consequences.

Consider the benefits of cholesterol discussed previously. Statin drugs undermine all of these benefits, resulting in side effects that erode the user's health:

1. There is a decline in the production of your adrenal and sex hormones with all the adverse effects of hormonal decline and imbalance.

2. Because cholesterol is essential for brain and nerve function, when it is lowered by statin drugs, patients often experience memory loss and even global amnesia.

3. There is an increased risk of liver disease and liver cancer. That is why your doctor will want you to come to his office for regular blood tests to check your liver enzymes if you are taking statin drugs.

4. Coenzyme Q10 (Co Q10), also known as ubiquinone, is essential for cellular production of energy, primarily in the heart and the liver. It is synthesized in the body, using the same pathway for

the synthesis of cholesterol. Statin drugs poison this biochemical pathway and dramatically inhibit the production of Co Q10.

5. Muscle pain and weakness are common side effects of statin drugs. This is caused by a condition known as rhabdomyolysis in which the muscles literally begin wasting away. Since your heart is a muscle, it is affected as well. For the elderly, muscle weakness and memory loss are especially debilitating side effects. These symptoms are usually viewed as signs of aging rather than the adverse side effects of statin drugs.

6. Statin drugs have also been shown to increase the risk for cancer, as has been revealed in the combination drug, Vytorin, which contains both the statin drug Zocor and also Zetia, which limits the absorption of cholesterol by the intestines. In the 1,873-patient SEAS study, the patients who took Vytorin developed twice as many cancers as the placebo group.

All of these side effects can accompany statin drug use, not to mention that your liver has to work harder to detoxify these chemicals from your body. The effects may not be immediate, but over a period of time these drugs have a compounding effect and begin to deteriorate your health. Considering that your chance of receiving a heart benefit from these drugs is only one or two in 100, the risks seem to outweigh the benefits.

Do statin drugs do what they are supposed to do? The answer is yes, they do lower cholesterol levels, but we have the wrong culprit. While Americans are busy lowering their cholesterol levels, the real thief is coming in through the back door.

COULD IT BE HYPOTHYROIDISM?

Heart disease may run rampant in your family, but there may be another reason underlying that familial trend, hypothyroidism. Hypothyroidism could be what is setting your family up to be victimized by heart disease. As we have discussed, prior to the use of antibiotics, Americans who suffered from hypothyroidism rarely survived childhood. These individuals succumbed to infectious disease in droves and were especially obliterated by tuberculosis. Meanwhile, Dr. Broda Barnes discovered that there was an inverse relationship between the rate of heart disease and tuberculosis among groups of people within certain regions.

Barnes was able to investigate this relationship further through a remarkable group for the study: the Graz autopsies. Because of a very high infant mortality in the city of Graz, Austria, in the late eighteenth century, Empress Marie Theresa of Austria mandated that autopsies be performed on every hospital death in Graz. The Graz autopsies became an incredible medical resource for physicians of the twentieth century and saved the lives of thousands through their findings.

CONVERGING LINES OF EVIDENCE

Dr. Barnes believed that hypothyroidism was related to heart disease before he began to study the Graz autopsies. Barnes had removed the thyroid glands of baby rabbits and found that their life spans were cut in half. They suffered from recurrent infections and accelerated arterial damage. Other physicians reported the same findings when they removed the thyroid glands of other animals for study. All found that upon the addition of thyroid hormone, the progression of atherosclerosis was stopped.

These findings along with his passion for hypothyroidism research inspired Dr. Barnes to travel to Austria each summer for more than 15 years to study the Graz autopsies. Dr. Barnes observed that the death rate from coronary artery disease in 1970 was ten times the death rate found in 1930. This is staggering considering that, statistically, the death rate would only be expected to double, certainly not be ten times the rate of coronary artery disease.

What could be the possible explanation? During this time period, life-saving antituberculin drugs and antibiotics saved the lives of thousands who would have otherwise perished from infectious diseases. Barnes observed this trend among epidemiological studies as well. The original populations, who had low rates of heart disease and were used as fodder to further the cholesterol theory, had high death rates from tuberculosis. Barnes found this trend reproduced in population after population: As the rates of death from tuberculosis dropped, so followed an increase in death from heart attacks.

Additional studies proved this link to be correct. The 2003 Rotterdam study demonstrated that subclinical hypothyroidism is an independent risk factor for heart atherosclerosis and myocardial infarction in elderly women.[63] Low thyroid function has been positively linked with an increased risk of heart disease. In 2008 the HUNT study found that women with a high TSH had a 69 percent increased rate of heart disease. This follows the assumption that as the TSH trends upward, thyroid production is declining.

TREATING HYPOTHYROIDISM AND HEART DISEASE

Does treating hypothyroidism lower the rate of heart disease? If so, the proof would be in the pudding. Getting to the bottom of this question was a key reason Dr. Barnes conducted the study described earlier in which he followed 1,569 of his patients treated for thyroid over the span of 8,824 patient years and found that only four new cases of cardiovascular disease were established—a 94 percent reduction in the anticipated incidence of the disease.

What is behind hypothyroidism's relationship with heart disease? The suspected culprit is mucin. Mucin is a normal part of our immune system that is present in our tissues and binds to pathogenic material in our body. In myxedema, or end-stage hypothyroidism, characterized by major swelling of the body, large levels of mucin are found. When mucin accumulates in the tissues abnormally, the result is swelling.

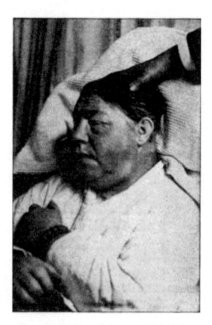

Source: Hertoghe, E. Medical Record, Sep. 1914, Vol.86, Issue 12, 489-505.

The swelling eventually spreads to all of your connective tissues. Mucin is responsible for the puffiness and water retention associated with hypothyroidism. The heart, which contains connective tissue, is seriously affected by hypothyroidism, and mucin leads to injury of the arteries. As tissues become engorged with mucin, heart function slows, which leads to a weak and wounded heart, unable to pump blood efficiently. It has been documented that treatment of an enlarged heart using natural thyroid supplementation reduces it to its normal size. Treatment with desiccated thyroid USP returns the tissues to normal, but if the treatment is halted, mucin again increases rapidly.

As you know, the thyroid is responsible for your body's metabolism. Normal thyroid metabolism helps to prevent recurrent infection and chronic inflammation. Your body's natural defense against inflammation is to produce antioxidants to fend off dangerous free radicals that create oxidative damage in your body. A slow metabolism not only affects the efficiency of the central nervous system, cardiovascular and skeletal systems, and kidneys and hormone producing tissues, it also affects the rate at which antioxidants are produced. The result is that few antioxidants are left to minimize the effects of free radicals. This leaves your arteries and blood vessels open to further attack, leading to atherosclerosis.

While Americans are busy worrying about their cholesterol levels and swallowing statin drugs with sugary soft drinks, the unsuspected killer is left to wreak havoc on American hearts. It saddens me to think of how many early deaths could have been prevented with proper assessment and treatment of hypothyroidism. As Dr. Barnes stated, "The first symptom of hypothyroidism that a patient may notice is a heart attack." If heart disease runs in your family, don't allow it to continue to affect you or your family members. If you have the symptoms of hypothyroidism and a low basal body temperature, it is imperative that you ask your physician for a therapeutic trial of natural desiccated thyroid USP. Your heart depends on it.

SUMMARY

1. Heart disease became a leading cause of death after antibiotics lowered the mortality rate from tuberculosis.

2. While more people are living long enough to develop heart disease, the prevalence of heart disease has remained unchanged since the turn of the century.

3. A relationship exists between hypothyroidism and elevated cholesterol levels.

4. Cholesterol is essential to health and plays many important roles in the body.

5. Using cholesterol-lowering drugs to prevent coronary artery disease is misguided.

6. Statin drugs have many significant adverse side effects and minimal benefits.

7. Treatment with desiccated thyroid hormone has been shown to lower the risk of heart attack.

8. For more information, please visit www.hotzehwc.com/CholesterolMyths.

chapter
SIX

OBESITY AND HYPOTHYROIDISM

hen I was a child, obesity was more the exception than the rule. There might have been that one kid in class who was considered chubby, but this was not very common. Fast forward 50 years to today. Seventy-seven percent of our children are overweight and 17 percent are obese. American children have increased their weight at the rate of 300 percent since 1980. This is not just an image problem or a concern of fitting into a certain mold set by society. Considering that being obese or just overweight dramatically increases the risk for the notorious American serial killers—high blood pressure, diabetes, heart disease, stroke, and cancer—this is a matter of life or death. Approximately 300,000 deaths per year in the United States are attributable to obesity. A study conducted between 2001 and 2004 demonstrated that two out of three Americans are overweight or obese. *Sixty-six percent of Americans are overweight and 34 percent are obese.*

THE EFFECTS OF OUR NATION'S HABIT

America's upward trending waistlines are increasingly evident in today's culture. America is becoming increasingly comfortable with being fat. Obesity has made its way into pop culture with television shows such as *The Biggest Loser*, further highlighting how mainstream the problem has become. The American marketplace has stretched to fit our bulging bodies and now products such as seatbelt extenders, jumbo umbrellas, extra large coat hangers, 96-inch tape measures for sewing, and special hygiene equipment for oversized Americans are becoming increasingly commonplace. The medical industry has had to make adjustments as well, from the smallest changes such as larger blood-pressure cuffs to bigger items such as 500-pound scales. Severe obesity shortens an individual's lifespan by 10 years and is comparable to a lifetime of smoking. To meet the growing demand, coffin companies have expanded their lines to include extra large and supersize coffins. The disease that characterized them in life now follows obese Americans into death.

Obesity is the result of a variety of factors such as our thyroid status, genetics, diet, and hormonal imbalance. Any one of these factors, combined with America's insatiable appetite and sedentary lifestyle, create a sort of Bermuda Triangle of disease, inescapable and deadly. For the overweight, current medicine offers the predictable answer: eat less and exercise more. But what if you are already doing this? Many Americans feel they could exercise seven days a week, eat a piece of celery for each meal, and still gain five pounds. For these individuals, mainstream medicine's only solutions are prescription drugs or surgery. This is a disservice to individuals struggling with this problem. We now know that obesity is not solely the result of eating too much and exercising too little. For many, being overweight is a result of a sluggish metabolism caused by hypothyroidism.

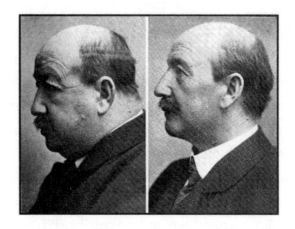

Source: Hertoghe, E. Medical Record, Sep. 1914, Vol.86, Issue 12, 489-505.

STRAIN ON THE MEDICAL SYSTEM

In 2008 the medical costs of obesity-related drugs in the United States skyrocketed to $147 billion, increasing $73 billion during the last decade.[64] If the trend continues, by 2018 it is estimated that 43 percent of Americans will be obese, resulting in an annual medical bill of obesity-related disease to be somewhere in the neighborhood of $343 billion. In 2008 obese people spent $1,429 more per person on medical costs than those with a normal weight.

CLINICAL HYPOTHYROIDISM AND OBESITY

As we discussed in previous chapters, gaining weight and the inability to lose weight are key symptoms of hypothyroidism. Many hypothyroid individuals have a very low metabolism. We have mentioned that a major indicator for hypothyroidism is a low basal body temperature. Let's discuss why this is an accurate measure of hypothyroidism.

The regulation of your metabolism is an elegant system in which your body functions because of a beautifully designed and complex series of biochemical reactions. You may remember from biology class that these biochemical reactions are catalyzed by specific enzymes.

Recall from Chapter 2 that there are two main thyroid hormones: triiodothyronine (T3), the active hormone and thyroxine (T4), the inactive thyroid hormone. Thyroxine (T4) must be converted into triiodothyronine (T3) in order to be used in your cells. There is a receptor site on each one of your cells made just for T3. Think of these receptor sites as keyholes by which T3, and only T3, gains entry into your cells to be used for energy. Your body can also convert T4 into another thyroid hormone, reverse T3 (RT3). RT3 has no other function in your cells other than blocking the T3 receptor sites, preventing T3 from entering into your cells. Normally, the amount converted into RT3 is so small there is enough T3 floating around to dominate and keep the balance in favor of T3. This is of course, if everything is normal within your body and, as we have discussed, we do not live in a perfect world.

For example, when the body is under stress, it initially begins to produce high amounts of cortisol to compensate. High amounts of cortisol block the conversion of T4 to T3 and favor the conversion of T4 to RT3. The result is that little active thyroid hormone, T3, is produced and the receptor sites are increasingly blocked by RT3. We've also seen how estrogen dominance, or progesterone deficiency, can also cause hypothyroidism, which can lead to weight gain and obesity.

─────────────────── **WORD WISE** ───────────────────

Obesity. Gradations of excessive body fat and weight are generally measured using body mass index, or BMI, a value that reflects appropriate weight associated with a given height. A normal BMI is 18.5 to 24.9;

overweight is 25 to 29.9, and obese is 30 and above. A person who is 5'9" would be considered overweight at 169 pounds and obese at 203 pounds. Though it's a standard measure, BMI isn't perfect, as it doesn't account for fitness or muscle mass.

ELLEN'S STORY

Ellen humorously describes herself as a 39-year-old business professional of relatively sound mind and body. However, she had endured a six-and-a-half-year personal nightmare to be able to say that.

At the young age of 33, Ellen felt as if a switch in her body had been thrown. She started feeling fatigued and lost all sexual desire. She knew that this shouldn't be happening at her age. When she arrived home from work, she would prepare a quick meal and do a little washing and cleaning so she could go to bed and get to sleep by 7:30 or 8:00 p.m. every night. She soon stopped exercising or engaging in any strenuous activities because of her severe fatigue.

Over the next year, Ellen gained an incredible 65 pounds. She began experiencing problems with her memory. She couldn't remember details of meetings she had attended in the morning by the time the afternoon rolled around. To compensate for this, she began taking extensive notes during every meeting to which she could later refer. She even developed her own version of "business appropriate" shorthand to try and capture every word possible during her meetings. This was the only method she had to help her remember her project assignments.

MEDICAL RUNAROUND

Ellen spoke to her ob/gyn at length about her symptoms during her annual visit. Condescendingly, her doctor told her, "You need to learn to deal with stress in ways other than using the refrigerator. Stop eating all that bread and dessert." Ellen was dumbfounded. She had just communicated what she thought were valid problems, and felt completely dismissed. She thought to herself, "I do like bread, but not enough to cause a weight gain of 65 pounds! As for dessert, cake at family-celebrated birthdays alone wouldn't cause the weight gain I experienced." At this stage she thought, "I'm not the crazy one; I have a doctor with the wrong attitude." Ellen found a new ob/gyn for her next annual visit.

Another year passed and Ellen's health continued to decline. Because of her family history for hypothyroidism, at her request, she was blood-tested twice for this condition. Her new doctor insisted that her blood tests were "normal" and there was "no problem" with her thyroid. Her physician warned her that her continued research and study about the symptoms for hypothyroidism was turning her into a hypochondriac. Initially, Ellen rejected his comments, but slowly she began to doubt herself.

SPIRALING SYMPTOMS

During this time, Ellen decided to try to get pregnant. When nothing happened, she and her husband were referred to a new ob/gyn, who also tested Ellen's thyroid, felt it was in a normal range, and diagnosed her as being depressed. Her health continued its downward spiral. She had developed severe PMS symptoms: fluid retention, moodiness, and severe headaches, which she experienced ten days out of each month. She had brittle, flaky fingernails; stiff, achy joints; dry skin; and painful, swollen breasts. She stated that her tongue was so swollen that she would awaken each night, choking. She was always cold, so much so that she slept in flannel night clothes with an electric blanket year round.

Ellen consulted with an infertility specialist who was an endocrinologist, reputed to be one of the best in the country. She was sure that this doctor would finally be the one who could piece together the puzzle of her symptoms and discover her problem. Her hopes were dashed when, after he too had tested her thyroid blood levels, he told her that they were "barely" within the normal range, but that this was "not a problem." Because Ellen was being evaluated for infertility, she was instructed to chart her body temperature for several months. She was told to buy a basal thermometer. This is a thermometer used to help predict ovulation, but it only starts measuring body temperature at 97 degrees. Ellen became frustrated because the thermometer would never register. Convinced it was broken, she exchanged it for a regular thermometer only to find that her body temperature was consistently lower than 97 degrees.

NO ANSWERS

The doctor's answer to all of this was to prescribe Parlodel. Parlodel is a fertility drug that was supposed to cause her to ovulate. Ellen continued to question the doctor as to why her body was not functioning properly. During the seven months that Ellen was taking Parlodel, she had two emergency room visits for shortness of breath and an accelerated heart rate. Ellen told me of one of those visits: "There's nothing in the world like overhearing the ER doctor describe you to the next doctor coming on shift as an 'obese female' in room 3. I cried until I fell asleep in the ER room and was later released."

Ellen found herself feeling so helpless that she would just start crying without any provocation several times a day. When she was home, she spent her time alternately crying and sleeping. Her confidence had been destroyed, and she doubted her sanity for "imagining" how miserable she felt.

Ellen's hair became so dry and brittle that she decided to have it cut short. This revealed that she had numerous bald spots. Her hair had been falling out at an alarming rate. She had also become so constipated that she could easily go eight days without a bowel movement. At work she began using her lunch hour to nap in her office because of her severe fatigue.

FINAL STRAW

At Ellen's insistence, her infertility specialist begrudgingly agreed to perform one more thyroid test to "humor" her. When he called her with the results, she was at home because she had taken a vacation day due to her tiredness. The doctor proceeded to tell her that she did not have a thyroid problem. He recommended to Ellen that she should seek the help of a mental health professional because he couldn't treat her anymore if she kept insisting her symptoms were related to thyroid problems. Incredibly, he told her that she wasn't tired but likely just lazy.

Ellen snapped! She yelled two words at him over the phone which I will not repeat and slammed the receiver down. Her doctor had just dismissed her as his patient and had insulted her while doing it. This interaction had caused her to feel dehumanized. There was no more safety raft to hold onto, and she was drowning in hopelessness. This was the bottom of the barrel. What she considered as her last chance to restore her life had just been ripped from her heart.

FINDING THE RIGHT TRACK

When Ellen came to the Hotze Health & Wellness Center one February morning, Dr. Sheridan listened to her saga without any demeaning comments. Instead he explained that her story was similar to that of thousands of other women whom he had successfully treated. Ellen felt vindicated by her long-awaited diagnosis of hypothyroidism. She also discovered the dramatic role her other hormones had played in the steep decline of her health. Knowing that this was her opportunity to get her life back, she gladly agreed to the treatment recommendations that she was offered.

By the end of the first week on the treatment program Ellen knew things were moving in the right direction. Within a month her coworkers could tell a difference. Her boss told her, "For the first time in a long time, I can see a sparkle in your green eyes." Steadily Ellen regained her energy, her drive, and her desire to engage in life. Within eight months she had lost 60 pounds and resolved the host of health symptoms and issues that she had been enduring for more than six years.

Thyroid is not a weight loss supplement. However, if not enough of this vital hormone gets into the cells, the metabolism slows down, which often contributes to weight gain. For Ellen, her eating habits were not the problem, but for many Americans, a junk food diet is a potentially life-threatening issue.

CREATING A FEEDING FRENZY

There is no doubt that America has an eating problem. As a nation, we are overfed and undernourished. Over the past 50 years the kind of food that most Americans consume and the amount they consume has dramatically changed. Combine the unrestricted availability of high calorie, processed, fast foods with a busy lifestyle and the result is a dietary disaster.

Who has time to cook dinner while simultaneously climbing the corporate ladder and picking kids up from soccer practice? The fast food industry has been more than willing to take advantage of this situation.

HOOKED ON FAST FOOD

Each day, one out of four Americans will eat at a fast food res-
taurant. Our spending reflects our addiction. In 2002 Americans spent
around $110 billion on fast food. McDonald's golden arches are now
more recognized than the Christian cross.

PROBLEMS WITH OFFICIAL RECOMMENDATIONS

Our diet is high in carbohydrates and low in nutrients. Part of this unbalanced diet is due to the United States Department of Agriculture's misguided food pyramid that people have used as a guide for decades.[65] The fact that grains had comprised the largest portion of the food pyramid comes as no surprise when you realize that the grain lobbies are among the most aggressive lobbying powers in government. Instead of developing a food guide that would enhance the health of the American public, a government-promoted food pyramid has been devised for the financial health of the U.S. agricultural lobbies representing grains, dairy, and meat. As a result, our nation has built a faulty food foundation for sound health. Next, the FDA released an updated plate approach. While grains are no longer the largest portion of the diet, bread still makes up more than one fourth of the plate. Milk is prominently displayed, although many Americans have an allergy to dairy products.

HEFTY PORTIONS AND CHEMICAL ADDITIVES

In this land of abundance, portion sizes have also increased. We have David Wallerstein, a theater chain manager, to thank for the larger portions, bigger drinks, and huge plates. Charged with increasing sales, Wallerstein discovered that people would gladly pay more for larger drinks and popcorn to avoid disrupting their movie with a trip to the concession stand. Thus was born the concept of the supersize. Wallerstein eventually became an executive at McDonald's, where his supersize idea found its wings. Americans were challenged to supersize everything under the golden arches, and the trend caught on in other areas of the food industry as well.

Around this same time, food manufacturers began experimenting with food additives. Monosodium glutamate, high-fructose corn syrup, aspartame, and many additional chemical preservatives became industry staples. These chemicals were designed to titillate the taste buds and induce cravings, and they did just that. Americans craved more food. Your liver treats these "foods" as chemicals and must detoxify each from your body. The chemicals tend to accumulate in your fat cells, leaving overweight individuals to store more food-chemical additives.

OBESITY AND ADDITIONAL HORMONES

Thyroid hormone is not the only hormone that plays a role in your metabolism. Because all of your hormones are intended to work together harmoniously, an imbalance or decline in just one hormone can create disharmony in the rest of your hormones.

As I have written earlier, in women, estrogen dominance causes the liver to produce thyroid-binding proteins that attach to the thyroid hormones and prevent them from being assimilated by your cells. Additionally, fat cells actually produce estrogen, not only perpetuating the cycle but also increasing your risk for cancer. It is important to note that estrogen is not bad in and of itself, but rather, estrogen unbalanced with progesterone produces the problem.[66] As women age, progesterone levels fall significantly faster than estrogen levels, creating an imbalance. Unopposed estrogen is what increases the risk for cancer.

Our environment increasingly plays a role in our risk for estrogen dominance as well. Not only are hormones found in our meat and dairy supply but estrogenic compounds contaminate many of our household products. These are called xenoestrogens, which are petrochemical compounds that exert estrogenic effects and hormonal dysfunction in both women and men. They leak into our foods through plastic containers and in personal hygiene and cleaning products.

In males, the inevitable decline in testosterone can lead to a decreased metabolism and an increased weight gain, especially around the belly. Have you ever noticed how many middle-aged men look as if they are wearing an inner tube? You can thank a decline in testosterone for that. And as we just learned, the more fat cells you have, the more estrogen you produce. The excess fat is why men often have increased levels of estrogen as they age.

Excess weight can cause an increase in estrogen in both women and men, which in turn leads to the growth of fat cells. This is a circular loop that perpetuates itself. Excess fat also causes insulin resistance, leptin resistance, and elevated blood sugar, high blood pressure, and decreased thyroid activity in the cells due to an increase in TBG.

OBESITY AND DIABETES

It is estimated that 80 percent of type 2 diabetes is related to obesity. In the next 25 years, the number of Americans with diabetes is projected to double from 24 million in 2009 to 48 million in 2034. But the existing situation is already bad enough, with 35 percent of adults over the age of 20, approximately 80 million Americans, currently having prediabetes, based upon their blood tests.

Diabetes is a leading cause of kidney damage, heart disease, stroke, blindness, and amputations caused by infections of the legs and feet. Statistically, diabetes is the cause of, or a contributing cause of, death in more than 600,000 Americans every year. This takes into account the underreporting of diabetes on death certificates. The average medical expenditures among people who had a diabetes diagnosis in 2007 were 2.3 times higher than medical expenditures for those who did not. According to research conducted by the Centers for Disease Control and Prevention (CDC) and the American Diabetes Association (ADA), the total cost of diagnosed diabetes in the United States in 2007 was $174 billion.[67] Yes, the American diet is loaded with sugar and simple carbohydrates and, yes, America is overweight, but 24 million people with diabetes? Is something else contributing to the rising incidence of type 2 diabetes? Let's take a look.

HOOKING TWO "HYPOS"

In order for your body to function normally, it requires a certain level of sugar or glucose, which is regulated by the hormone, insulin, made by your pancreas. When your blood sugar rises, the pancreas releases insulin to cause the cells to utilize the sugar in the blood, lowering your sugar level. Hypoglycemia means low blood sugar or glucose. Common factors leading to hypoglycemia are large amounts of refined carbohydrates in the diet, allergies, and hypothyroidism.[68]

During his research, Dr. Broda Barnes found that the incidence of hypoglycemia is much lower when patients are treated with thyroid. This would suggest that hypoglycemia correlates with hypothyroidism. In addition, the thyroid has a profound effect on the liver, which can also lower blood glucose levels.

Thyroid problems occur more often in people with diabetes. One reason is that when the antibodies attack the thyroid gland, you may have a higher risk of your immune system attacking another endocrine gland. In type 1 diabetes, antibodies attack the islet cells of the pancreas, decreasing the production of insulin.

A person with hypothyroidism may be at risk for metabolic syndrome or insulin resistance, both of which could lead to type 2 diabetes. Research correlates autoimmune thyroiditis to type 1 diabetes.[69] It is critical that diabetic patients receive a regular thyroid checkup.

The average medical expenditures among people who had a diabetes diagnosis in 2007 were 2.3 times higher than medical expenditures for those who did not.

OBESITY AND HIGH BLOOD PRESSURE

One in three Americans has high blood pressure, an estimated 74,500,000 adults in the United States. Approximately 69 percent of people who have had their first heart attack, 77 percent of those who have had their first stroke, and 74 percent of those who have had coronary heart failure have high blood pressure. Twenty-six percent of obese individuals have high blood pressure. Is it the obesity alone that is causing the high blood pressure or is high blood pressure, like obesity, a symptomatic offspring of the same parent?

The relationship between hypothyroidism and high blood pressure has been noted in several American journals. Dr. Broda Barnes observed this relationship among his hypothyroid patients more than 50 years ago, noting that as the patient was treated with natural desiccated thyroid, the blood pressure began to normalize.

This connection between high blood pressure and hypothyroidism lies in the kidneys. The kidneys are especially hit hard by hypothyroidism, resulting in decreased blood flow and circulation. When blood flow is diminished in the kidneys, they produce a hormone called renin, which increases blood pressure. Rather than treating the root issue, doctors are busy treating the symptom with antihypertensive medications, calcium channel blockers, ACE inhibitors, beta blockers, and diuretics. They may lower your blood pressure, but at what cost? These drugs come with a long list of side effects such as dizziness, heart palpitations, insomnia, kidney damage, loss of taste, fatigue, decreased mental sharpness, and impotence, to name a few. Upon reviewing the results of thyroid treatment for blood pressure, shouldn't we treat the underlying cause rather than continue to mask the symptoms?

THE RESULT OF OBESITY-RELATED ILLNESS

Obesity is related to the top diseases affecting the American population. In addition to diabetes, blood pressure, and hypertension, 42 percent of breast and colon cancers were diagnosed among the American obese population, and 30 percent of gallbladder surgery is directly related to obesity. Seventy percent of cardiovascular disease is related to obesity. With obesity also comes an increased risk for osteoarthritis, sleep apnea, and depression.

Obesity in and of itself takes a toll on one's personal psyche. Being involved in activities becomes increasingly difficult and uncomfortable. Eventually, your job is affected when tasks that require working beyond the confines of a desk remain undone. Your social life begins to wane. By far, the toll that obesity takes on your family and loved ones hurts the most. It may begin slowly. You are unable to keep up with your child practicing soccer so you watch from the sidelines. You decline invitations to family birthday parties. You miss your child's swim meet. The progression is slow, but you find yourself checking out of life. Maybe you are like many Americans whose weight crept up on them. You may have tried dieting and exercising without favorable results, so you gave up. If this is the case, I encourage you to continue watching what you eat and get plenty of exercise but consider the possibility that, like Ellen, your thyroid hormone function may not be optimal. By correcting a thyroid imbalance, you can cut the knot that binds you to a life predisposed to obesity, diabetes, high blood pressure, cancer, and heart disease.

SUMMARY

1. Obesity and weight gain have become a way of life for the majority of Americans.
2. Metabolism plays a major role in the body's weight regulation.
3. Fast food, oversized portions, misguided dietary recommendations, and food additives also play a role in this epidemic.
4. Obesity is closely tied to major chronic diseases including type 2 diabetes and high blood pressure.
5. Treating hypothyroidism can alleviate weight problems.
6. For more information, please visit www.hotzehwc.com/ ObesityEpidemic.

chapter
SEVEN

POLYPHARMACY AND HYPOTHYROIDISM

MARY'S MOTHER'S STORY

Mary is a guest at my center who shared with me her concern and anger at the lack of care that her mother had received. After being diagnosed with cancer, Mary's mother initially did well on her own. When things started taking a turn for the worse, Mary moved in to care for her. As she began to look over her mother's affairs and assess the situation, she discovered that her mother was religiously taking 26 different medications every day. Alarmed, Mary began to research each drug. To her horror, she found that half of them counteracted the other drugs that she was taking. Mary's mother was fortunate that she had an advocate in her daughter. Many elderly are not so fortunate. Sadly, this scenario is not an isolated event and highlights an ever-increasing and dangerous trend in America.

AN AMERICAN AFFAIR WITH DRUGS

The United States spends more on prescription drugs than any other industrialized nation in the world. Death from prescription drugs is the second cause of unintentional death in the United States, second only to motor vehicle crashes. The number of people poisoned by prescription drugs has increased by at least 20,000 each year since 2008, with 82,724 deaths in 2010.[70] We're not talking about illegal narcotics, but rather doctor-prescribed, FDA-approved drugs. Of even greater concern is that this number is on the rise. The baby boomer generation saw an increase of 90 percent in prescription drug deaths. Sadly, the age group that has made the biggest jump in prescription drug deaths was among the ages of 15 to 24 years. According to the CDC, this is due to the recreational use of legally prescribed drugs. This type of use of prescription drugs is a gateway to the use of illegal drugs, such as cocaine and methamphetamine, in the future. We are telling our children to say, "Just say no!" to illegal drugs, but ironically we are desensitizing them to drug use at an early age.

In every one of their television advertisements, pharmaceutical companies are telling Americans to "Just say yes!" to drugs.

What has also become increasingly more American is the practice of polypharmacy, patients being on multiple drugs at one time. A recent study analyzing data from 13,000 psychiatric office visits, found that the percentage of visits in which two or more psychiatric medications were prescribed, such as antidepressants and antianxiety drugs, increased from 43 percent in 1996 to 60 percent a decade later. In addition, visits in which three or more drugs were prescribed rose from 17 percent in 1996 to 33 percent in 2006. These are just the psychiatric medications. This does not include sleep aids, high blood pressure medications, cholesterol-lowering drugs, anti-inflammatories, and a mountain of other drugs for gastrointestinal problems, urinary difficulty, impotency, weight loss, hair loss, allergies, and so on.

> *Death from prescription drugs is the second largest cause of unintentional death in the United States, second only to motor vehicle crashes.*

UNNECESSARY OVERMEDICATION

You might be thinking, "So what does polypharmacy have to do with hypothyroidism?" The answer is that it is not a cause of hypothyroidism but, rather, the result of unrecognized and untreated hypothyroidism by many medical doctors. Think of the drug advertisements you watch on television or read on the pages of glossy magazines, in newspapers, and on banner ads on the Internet. They are touting treatments for fatigue, weight gain, constipation, gastroesophageal reflux, insomnia, depression, migraines, impotence, joint and muscle pain, and elevated cholesterol, just to name a few. Look closer. Ask yourself, "What can cause each of these symptoms for which these multitude of drugs are prescribed? These are all symptoms of hypothyroidism! Mainstream medicine appears to be unable to see past the symptoms to the underlying cause. Instead of treating the root problem, hypothyroidism, mainstream doctors continue to mask the symptoms with prescription drugs. Remember, prescription drugs are associated with serious and harmful side effects.

If you continue down the pathway of current medicine, you will find yourself faced with the problem of polypharmacy.

Here's another sign of America's love affair with prescription drugs: Americans make up just 5 percent of the world's population, yet we consume 42 percent of all pharmaceutical drugs. In 2011 Americans spent $310 billion on prescription drugs.

AMERICA'S TOP-SELLING DRUG CLASSES

You may be surprised to learn that the United States and New Zealand are the only two countries where direct-to-consumer advertisement of prescription drugs is allowed. Driven in part by this advertising, here's what patients buy most:

- Cholesterol-lowering drugs, called statins by most people, the top-seller being Lipitor;
- Antidepressants. The selective-serotonin reuptake inhibitors, or SSRI, are the most popular, but a range of drugs are used in an attempt to correct mood, sleep, and concentration in depressed patients;
- Narcotic analgesics, also known as pain medications;
- Beta blockers. These drugs lower blood pressure by blocking norepinephrine and epinephrine, thereby reducing the heart rate;
- ACE inhibitors. These drugs also lower blood pressure, but by dilating blood vessels.

THE INFLUENCE OF ADVERTISING

Why has this happened? Were you aware that the average American watches 16 hours of drug advertisements on television every year? Have you ever been watching your favorite television show with your family when suddenly the show cuts to a commercial break that turns out to be an advertisement for a drug that treats impotency? This is probably not the kind of commercial that you want your children or grandchildren to view. Have you wondered how it has come to be that drug companies can advertise on television? Well, you can thank the Food and Drug Administration (FDA) for that.[71]

For years the drug companies licked their chops over the possibility of advertising on television. They knew that this would dramatically increase the sales of drugs, but the FDA had strict rules that prevented television advertising. The FDA had required a detailed list of side effects and contraindications to be reported. While this could be done in magazine advertisements, there was just not enough time to list all the side effects of drugs in a 30-second television commercial.

Then, in 1997, the FDA relaxed its rules, after strong lobbying by the Pharmaceutical Research and Manufacturers of America, commonly known as Big Pharma. The FDA decided that it would now allow drug companies to simply state a few of the side effects and then tell consumers to ask their physicians for more information. This was a boon to pharmaceutical sales, and the drug companies started spending money hand over fist to convince consumers to buy their products. The pharmaceutical industry spent more than $4.8 billion on direct-to-consumer advertising in 2011, $2.3 billion on television ads alone. This has paid off handsomely for Big Pharma. In 2008 the largest drug companies generated approximately $500 billion in gross revenues and $110 billion in profits.

This advertising is geared not only to you, the consumer, but to medical professionals as well.

PITCHING POLYPHARMACY

You've seen the drug commercials on television, full of happy people, having the time of their lives because they are taking the latest drug. The commercials imply or state outright that if you really want to enjoy life, you must take their drug. If you believe the commercials, by taking antidepressants, you can have the sun shining in your heart all the time. If the antidepressants do not work, you can add the new antipsychotic drug, Abilify, to your drug cocktail. If you are having trouble sleeping, you can buy a good night's rest with Ambien or Lunesta. That little Lunesta butterfly seems so gentle that it must surely make you float off into a sound sleep and wake up feeling refreshed. If you have joint and muscle aches, there are a host of anti-inflammatories to ease the pain, some of which, like Vioxx, dramatically increase your risk of dying from a heart attack. Vioxx was finally banned by the FDA in 2004.

If pharmaceutical companies do one thing well, it's marketing. They have managed to make prescription drugs seem like a normal part of life. This is no small feat. In 2008 pharmaceutical companies spent an unbelievable $4.8 billion on direct-to-consumer television, radio, magazine, and newspaper advertising.[72] This is twice what drug companies spend for research and development, but the payoffs are enormous. Just look at Pfizer's blockbuster drug Lipitor, for which sales in 2008 neared $13 billion. If Lipitor was actually making a huge dent in the rate of heart disease, it might be worth it. However, its effects on reducing heart disease are minimal and come with a host of many serious side effects.

In 2008 pharmaceutical companies spent $4.8 billion on direct-to-consumer television, radio, magazine, and newspaper advertising. This is twice what drug companies spend for research and development.

PRESCRIBING UNDER THE INFLUENCE

Have you ever wondered where your physician gets the latest information regarding the drug you were just prescribed? Do you think that he or she pores over scientific journals and research to determine the best drug for you? Unfortunately, that is not the way that our current medical system is set up, nor is there time for your doctor to stay up to date on the ever-changing landscape of pharmaceutical drugs. By and large, physicians get their information regarding the latest drugs from pharmaceutical sales representatives and from television advertisements.

You probably think that pharmaceutical sales representatives must have degrees in biochemistry or backgrounds in scientific research. Wrong. Most pharmaceutical sales representatives have backgrounds in sales, business, and communications. If you think that pharmaceutical sales are about educating the doctors and the public, you are sorely mistaken. Pharmaceutical companies are all about sales.[73]

When I started in practice in 1977, almost all the pharmaceutical drug representatives were middle-aged men, but times have changed. Now, pharmaceutical sales representatives are usually attractive young women with engaging personalities who excel in the power of persuasion. The drug companies know how to get your doctor's attention. This is not to say that pharmaceutical sales representatives are purposefully misleading doctors. I am sure many of you know someone in pharmaceutical sales and cannot imagine her being sly or deceptive. Often, these sales representatives are just as misled by their companies as are the doctors who receive their misrepresented statistics and their misguided sales pitch.

Their job is to present the information in a way that flatters the drug. They usually visit a physician's office by bringing complimentary lunch for the whole staff and leave behind a plethora of drug samples and a trail of pens with their drug's logo. Notice the pens, pads, and medical paraphernalia that are emblazoned with drug logos the next time you visit any physician's office, other than mine. At my office, pharmaceutical sales representatives are not allowed through the doors.

SIDE EFFECTS AND PROFITS

Part of the problem with polypharmacy is that the drugs and their effects have not been tested with other drugs that might be prescribed simultaneously to the same individual. The elderly seem to suffer from this the most because their care is often managed by several doctors, and often, nursing homes. Each doctor is often not fully aware of the medications the other doctors have prescribed. The common story is that a drug is given to relieve a symptom. Along with that drug comes a particular side effect for which a subsequent drug is given. This story repeats itself over and over in the lives of tens of millions of individuals. The patient who originally complained of one or more symptoms may wind up with multiple medications to relieve the additional symptoms caused by various medications she is taking.

You have seen the drug advertisements on television with beautiful people smiling and laughing as they jog down the beach. A soothing and competent voiceover recites a list of the side effects that the drug might cause: dizziness, vomiting, hair loss, loss of libido, blindness, cancer, hemorrhages, and an increased risk of suicide. If you let yourself be fooled by the drug companies, you may find yourself blind, hemorrhaging, afflicted with cancer, oblivious to your spouse, and on suicide watch, feeling worse than you did before you visited your doctor for help.

Tamoxifen, for example, a drug prescribed to women who have been diagnosed with breast cancer, falls into this category. Many of those poor women died of uterine cancer instead of breast cancer.[74]

It is only noted that the patient did not die of breast cancer. You probably would agree with me that if the patient dies, the treatment was not a success.

PATIENTS VERSUS PAYOFF

Pharmaceutical companies, like life insurance companies, are publicly traded businesses listed on the stock exchanges. Their primary purpose is to make a profit. While this may be good for the stockholders, it is not always in the best interest of patients. These companies are solely interested in promoting the use of drugs to address health problems, despite the fact that drugs only treat the symptoms of illness and never address the underlying cause. Drugs are unnatural chemicals that have been made in pharmaceutical laboratories, and their use is usually accompanied by a host of adverse side effects. Remember that drugs must be detoxified by your body, and as you get older your body is less able to eliminate drug toxins.

As I have explained in the preceding chapters, illness is not caused by a lack of prescription drugs. Most illnesses are due to poor dietary habits and nutrition; lack of exercise; allergic disorders that weaken the immune system and make it more prone to infection and yeast overgrowth, due to overuse of antibiotics; an imbalance and decline in the body's production of thyroid and sex hormones; and stressed adrenal glands. All of these factors can be addressed safely, effectively, and naturally without drugs.

Physicians who obtain their continuing education at conferences sponsored by the drug companies are unaware of this because they are indoctrinated with the dogma being promoted by Big Pharma. Physicians are often too willing to believe whatever the drug companies tell them about a product's safety and effectiveness.

THE VIOXX CATASTROPHE

A recent example is the Vioxx debacle. Vioxx is a member of a new class of painkillers called COX-2 inhibitors, used to treat arthritis. Vioxx received a speedy approval from the FDA in 1999, but it was pulled from the market in October 2004 after it was shown to dramatically increase the risk of heart attacks in those who used it.[75] Merck, the maker of Vioxx, had been warned by researchers of this potential problem in 1998. Despite this, Merck released and promoted Vioxx to overly trusting physicians and to the public.

When pharmaceutical companies are sued for product liability because of the adverse side effects of their drugs, they claim that they cannot be held liable because their drugs have been approved by the Food and Drug Administration (FDA). It seems that the drug companies want to take all the benefit in terms of profits and leave the risk totally on the shoulders of the doctors and patients who have no recourse.

CONSTRAINTS ON HMOS

Physicians who are enrolled in health maintenance organizations have their hands tied when it comes to treatment. They must treat you by using the specific drugs that the HMO has approved, rather than with safer, natural therapies. To protect your health you simply must get out of HMOs and hire a doctor who will work for you rather than for the insurance companies or for the government.

AMERICA'S CHOICE

Most of the blame falls squarely on the shoulders of Big Pharma, but not all. After all, no one is forced to take pharmaceutical drugs, the exception being those who have been pronounced mentally incompetent and placed in a psychiatric ward. Parents in this country tell their kids to say no to drugs, but do they do as they say? Maybe it's time for adults to start leading by example.

It seems that many Americans just want a pill that can make the aches and pains and the troubles of the world go away. In an age of instant gratification, people are looking for an instant fix, a cure-all, a magic pill. The truth is that there isn't a pill in the world that can undo a lifetime of abuse to your body.

It's time for Americans to take charge of their own health and the first step is to kick the pharmaceutical drug habit. Prescription drugs have a place in medical care and treatment, but they are vastly overused. I believe physicians should treat along the lines of divine design, working with the body rather than against it. Our bodies were fearfully and wonderfully made. It's time we started treating them that way.

MARCIA'S STORY

"I would have been dead by now!" This is what Marcia believed to be true based upon the treatment she had been receiving at the hands of her physicians and the pharmaceutical drugs she had been consuming at their recommendation. This is her story, in her own words:

Postsurgical Symptoms

It all started in 1993, with a medical, surgical error of a gynecologist that caused major endometriosis and scar tissue growth after I had a hysterectomy. The doctor had to halt the surgery because everything inside my stomach was attached and he considered it too dangerous to continue at that time. Later, in 2002, through laparoscopy, the ovaries and scar tissue were removed.

After these surgeries, I thought my nightmare of feeling sick, muscle and joint pain, cognitive dysfunction, and horrible mood swings would be alleviated by taking the prescribed estradiol. I thought it put me on an even keel.

Two months later, I had my first panic attack. Over the next few months, these attacks increased and were accompanied with crippling depression and insomnia. Our family doctor prescribed Ambien, which would give me an hour [of] sleep. She gave me Zoloft, and after a week of not sleeping at all, not eating, and feeling nauseated, the suicidal thoughts came. I really did not want to live anymore. At that time these drugs did not come with a warning that they may cause suicidal thoughts.

Fateful Intervention

One morning, when I was too sick to drive to work, I planned my suicide and got ready to execute my plan when the phone rang. Automatically, I picked up. Nothing is coincidental. It was the doctor's nurse, asking me how I was doing. When she understood what was going on, she told me to call my husband and go to the emergency room. How unfortunate, because they put me in a psychiatric ward, where of course, I was given several drugs.

This was a different experience. I felt so bad for these poor people locked up in there and felt I did not belong there. I was released after two days and sent to a psychiatrist who, of course, put me on an antidepressant, Wellbutrin, and a tranquilizer, Klonopin.

Falling on Deaf Ears

My observation to every doctor that my mental state coincided with the hysterectomy fell on deaf ears. I went to several gynecologists, an endocrinologist, and three different psychiatrists. They doled out psychiatric drugs like candy. 'Here try this!' When upping the dose of Klonopin to 1 mg did not work, I refused to take bigger doses. One psychiatrist even told me I could take this drug for two years without a problem. As they say, 'Yeah, right.' After six months I was hooked. I have never taken any illegal drugs and always felt hesitant regarding prescribed medications.

An illustration of how little attention some of these doctors pay to their patients is when I was on my second or third visit with one of the psychiatrists. She walked in the room, saying, 'Oh, you are the one who hears voices in her head?' Never had I mentioned voices. It stunned me, especially when she prescribed a twin medication to Zoloft that sent me spiraling down into the suicidal thought abyss, after which she gave me 15 mg of Remeron.

Finding Help

I am amazed now that I did not lose my job or my husband during those years. It was very trying for my husband. I felt so bad for him and was grateful we did not have any children at home. My husband stood by my side, and even though he did not always understand what was going on, he always believed in me.

After stumbling another year through the fog of these drugs and still in pain and misery, I visited the Hotze Health & Wellness Center, where Dr. Sheridan confirmed my suspicions regarding the connection between hormones and the problems I was having. What a relief to look at the big picture—my entire body and mind and not just pieces.

I was diagnosed with hormonal imbalance, adrenal fatigue, clinical hypothyroidism, and yeast overgrowth. They instructed me regarding diet, exercise, hormonal treatment, and supplements. Of course, there was also the issue of weaning off the antidepressants and Klonopin.

Because of the weaning off Klonopin, Wellbutrin and Remeron, it has not been a walk in the park, to say the least. Some of these drugs reportedly are worse to get rid of than street drugs. Through their continued support, my determination to get well became stronger. Dr. Sheridan, the physician assistant, and the nurses would encourage me each time I would hit a very hard spot, reminding me how far I had already made it through.

Due to the medications I had been taking, recovery took a little longer for me than for most patients. Nevertheless, it has been worth it because every day is one step closer towards health and happiness.

A Message for Other Women

I wish I could reach out to all women so that they would not have to go on the treacherous path that I walked on. I have already encountered too many of them on antidepressants and tranquilizers, and too many of them not seeing a way out of their pain. Every time, I tell them of the good news, 'Yes, there is light at the end of the tunnel and you can get well.'

I am now at the very end of tapering off Remeron and feeling better every day. I am so happy I do not have to see the psychiatrist any more. I am so happy to feel happy again.

I am so happy that depression is now a thing of the past and the anxiety demon is gone too! I am so happy to be excited about the future at 51 years of age and my husband is so happy to have his good wife back.

MEDICAL PERSPECTIVE

Marcia's story has a happy ending, but I am always grieved and disturbed when I think about the tens of millions of other women who are experiencing the same ordeal that she did.

After Marcia's hysterectomy, the first prescription that she was given was an estrogen hormone, estradiol. Because her gynecologist did not balance her hormones with progesterone, Marcia was immediately thrown into a state of estrogen dominance. As we have discussed, one of the side effects of estrogen dominance is hypothyroidism. The numerous symptoms that she described can be easily mitigated by balancing the female hormones with appropriate amounts of bioidentical estrogen *and* progesterone, plus supplementing with desiccated thyroid USP. Unfortunately, because she wasn't prescribed these safe, natural products but instead was prescribed a polypharmacy cocktail of five or six mind-altering drugs, Marcia had to suffer through years filled with terrifying thoughts, declining health, and deteriorating relationships before finding a path to restore her health, transform her life, and improve her world, naturally.

Antidepressants and antianxiety drugs are some of the most dangerous pharmaceutical products on the market because of their harmful side effects and addictive natures. They are prescribed like candy by doctors who apparently give little or no thought to their harmful side effects.

ANTIDEPRESSANTS: A PUBLIC HEALTH DISASTER

Pharmaceutical companies have perpetrated an incredible fraud upon the medical profession and millions of patients through deceptive research, business practices, and advertising regarding the safety and effectiveness of antidepressants since the early 1990s.

This deception by the drug companies has been perpetrated on the American public with the collusion of the FDA. Millions of patients have suffered severe and debilitating side effects, even suicide, from the use of antidepressants or from withdrawal reactions that can occur with the discontinuation of these drugs. Antidepressants are addictive. This is what creates the withdrawal reactions seen in the vast majority of patients who try to stop using them.

There are two major classes of prominently used antidepressants: selective serotonin reuptake inhibitors (SSRI), such as Prozac, and the serotonin norepinephrine reuptake inhibitors (SNRI), such as Effexor. These antidepressants operate by the same biochemical mechanism as cocaine, which is a super neurotransmitter reuptake inhibitor. Cocaine boosts the levels of three neurotransmitters: serotonin, noradrenalin, and dopamine. Drug companies researched and developed drugs that mimic the effects of cocaine. Now you understand why antidepressants are addictive.

ANTIDEPRESSANT EXPLOSION

A recent 2011 report from the National Center for Health Statistics indicates that more than 10 percent, or 30 million Americans are on antidepressants. The current antidepressants are referred to as blockbuster drugs by the pharmaceutical companies for good reason: According to Reuters, in 2009, antidepressant sales reached $9.9 billion, making antidepressants the third leading class of drugs in sales revenue in the United States. All told, there has been a staggering 400 percent increase in the use of antidepressants between 1991 and 2010.

What's more, women are prescribed antidepressants three times more frequently than men. Nearly 30 percent of white women between the ages of 40 and 60 are taking antidepressants. This percentage increases as you move up the socioeconomic scale. At the Hotze Health & Wellness Center, approximately 75 percent of our new women guests who present to us for evaluation are on, or have been on, antidepressants, or have been prescribed antidepressants but refused to take them. Yet withdrawal side effects, which can be severe, occur in upwards of 78 percent of patients trying to discontinue antidepressants.

SIDE EFFECTS MINIMIZED

The serious side effects and the withdrawal reactions associated with discontinuing antidepressants clearly represent a public health disaster of enormous proportions.

Dr. Joseph Glenmullen's book, *The Antidepressant Solution*, has tremendously influenced my thinking on the dangers of antidepressants. Dr. Glenmullen is a clinical instructor in psychiatry at Harvard Medical School and is on the staff of the Harvard University Health Services. He has written and spoken extensively on the dangerous side effects caused by antidepressants, especially the withdrawal side effects.

For more than two decades, pharmaceutical companies have only reported positive studies about the use of antidepressants. They have denied any serious side effects caused by use of the antidepressants or withdrawal reactions when they are discontinued. As a matter of fact, the pharmaceutical companies have disingenuously adopted the terminology of "discontinuation symptoms" so that they can deny that there are withdrawal effects. Warning of withdrawal reactions would be an admission that antidepressants are addictive, a classification that the drug companies continue to deny.

Drug companies conduct their own studies, independent of the FDA, in an attempt to prove the statistically significant benefits of the drug. The pharmaceutical companies look at the results of the various studies and then design further research in such a way that they achieve two statistically positive studies. In order to grant its approval for a drug, the FDA only requires that two studies be submitted that show that there is a statistical difference between the drug being evaluated and a placebo.

The FDA does not require that the drug companies submit any studies that statistically demonstrate negative side effects. It does not matter whether the effects are clinically significant or not. This differs from the requirement of the British Medicines and Healthcare Products Regulatory Agency (MHRA), equivalent to our FDA, which requires that the drug companies submit all the studies, both positive and negative, for review.

A DIFFERENT VIEW OVERSEAS

The British MHRA has essentially banned the use of any antidepressants in children under 18 years of age. The MHRA evaluated all the drug companies' reports and determined that antidepressants had no positive effect for children. In fact, the MHRA determined that antidepressants were dangerous, and that they led to an increase in suicidal thoughts and actions.

The drug companies have been aware of the side effects and the withdrawal reactions associated with the antidepressants, but they have been more interested in the multibillion-dollar profits from antidepressant sales than in public safety. The pharmaceutical companies have done everything in their power to hide these negative studies from the public and from physicians.

BUYING GOOD PR

Drug companies also finance studies created by public relations researchers and ghostwriters to prove positive statistical results for antidepressants to submit to medical journals. These studies are then published under the name of influential academic physicians who are paid handsome fees for the use of their names.

Pharmaceutical companies have been exposed for paying academic physicians to produce positive studies and promote the companies' drugs to the medical community at large. Dr. Marcia Angell, former editor-in-chief of the prestigious *New England Journal of Medicine*, wrote a groundbreaking book, *The Truth about the Drug Companies: How They Deceived Us and What to Do about It*.[76] In it, Angell writes that the pharmaceutical companies not only use their enormous economic power to induce academic physicians to promote their products but also arrange consulting contracts with researchers at the FDA and National Institutes of Health (NIH) to do the same.

THE TWISTED ROAD OF PROZAC

Prozac received FDA approval in 1987. Within the first four years of its release, the FDA had been made aware by the public, by physicians, and through published medical reports that the risk of suicidal ideation and suicide had dramatically increased in patients taking Prozac. In September 1991, the FDA summoned a panel of so-called experts to investigate the concern of the public and physicians that Prozac use was leading to an increased incidence of suicides among users of the drug. The panel consisted of nine members, five of whom had financial ties to the pharmaceutical companies. There was clearly a conflict of interest present among the members. The committee voted six to three not to warn the public of the suicidal risk present with the use of Prozac. Given the makeup of the committee, this does not seem surprising. What is surprising is that three members had the courage to vote to issue the warning.

It was not until March 2004 that the FDA finally issued a warning that adult and pediatric patients on antidepressants could develop a range of side effects that may make them suicidal, including anxiety, agitation, panic attacks, insomnia, irritability, hostility, impulsivity, akathesia (severe restlessness) hypomania, and mania. The FDA further warned that patients are most vulnerable to suicide and these other side effects when the treatment is initiated, and when the dose is either increased or decreased. This FDA warning was due in large part to diligent efforts of Dr. Joseph Glenmullen who had been warning of the serious side effects of antidepressants for over a decade, and to his testimony at the 2004 FDA hearing. Then, in October 2004, the FDA required that a black box warning be added to all pharmaceutical information regarding the use of antidepressants in children. This warning stated that children and adolescents taking antidepressants are at an increased risk for suicidal thinking and actions. In May 2007 this black box warning was required to be added to antidepressant information in individuals from 18 to 24 years of age. Why did it take so long for the FDA to fulfill its mission to protect the public?

To combat the negative press, the drug companies that manufactured antidepressants had ghostwriters at public relations firms research and write articles that continued to extol the benefits of antidepressants. These articles were published under the names of prominent academic psychiatrists who were paid considerable sums for their influence. The articles were then disseminated to drug salesmen who were sent out to calm the concerns of practicing physicians, using this deceptive marketing plan.

> *The FDA finally issued a warning that adult and pediatric patients on antidepressants could develop a range of side effects that could make them suicidal.*

QUESTIONING EFFECTIVENESS

On February 19, 2012, CBS's *60 Minutes* program featured Irving Kirsch, professor of psychology at the University of Hull in the United Kingdom and author of *The Emperor's New Drugs: Exploding the Antidepressant Myth.* Kirsch was interviewed regarding his recently published data that demonstrates that antidepressants are no more effective than placebos in the treatment of depression. This report has the potential of rocking the medical world and dethroning antidepressants from their exalted position in the treatment of a host of symptoms.

Drug companies have preyed on physicians using deceptive research and marketing material for decades. They have indoctrinated the public to believe that antidepressants are a panacea for a host of problems by inundating the public with television commercials promoting their benefits. The drug companies have never warned physicians or the public about the addictive nature of antidepressants or the significant withdrawal reactions that attend the discontinuation of these drugs.

Drug companies have marketed antidepressants for the masses. They have expanded their recommendations for antidepressants to include not only depression, for which they are prescribed only 25 percent of the time, but also for anxiety, panic attacks, attention deficit disorder, insomnia, PMS, headaches, crowd phobia, lack of mental focus, and fatigue, just to name a few.

Primary physicians have been the main marketing focus of the pharmaceutical companies that manufacture antidepressants. Currently, 79 percent of patients are taking antidepressants that have been prescribed by their primary care doctors. Due to their heavy schedules, these physicians are extremely dependent upon the drug detailing provided by drug company representatives who, more and more, are attractive young women. Get the picture?

DIFFICULTY QUITTING

Not only are the side effects of antidepressants downplayed by the drug representatives to the doctors but, also, little or nothing is mentioned about the often-severe withdrawal reactions that occur when these drugs are discontinued.

The withdrawal reactions may be mild, moderate, or severe depending upon how long the antidepressant has been used and the strength of the dose.

Depending upon the half-life of the drug, the time that the drug takes to be eliminated from the body, withdrawal reactions can occur almost immediately, even when one dose is missed.

In his book, *The Antidepressant Solution,* Joseph Glenmullen, MD, details his 5-Step Antidepressant Tapering Program, which instructs physicians how to avoid uncomfortable or dangerous withdrawal reactions in their patients. This book should be required reading for any physicians who are currently prescribing antidepressants. This book should also be read by any individual who has been prescribed an antidepressant.

GUARD AGAINST DRUGS

Polypharmacy, the practice of prescribing multiple drugs for one patient, is equally dangerous. My goal is to give you the information about this common medical practice so that you can be on your guard and protect yourself. Drugs are dangerous. They are chemicals that have never existed before in nature and were created in pharmaceutical labs. Drugs are toxins that must be detoxified by your liver. Toxins are poisons. The use of multiple drugs is exponentially dangerous. You and you alone are responsible for your health, and the sooner you take charge of it, the better off you will be. You may lose it forever if you let others, especially physicians, make the decisions for you.

This reminds me of what my dad often told me when I initially began my practice, "Don't poison your patients with all those drugs like the other doctors do." Dad was a successful entrepreneur who was gifted with common sense. I am glad that I finally followed his advice.

QUESTIONS TO ASK YOUR DOCTOR

Any time a physician prescribes a medication, you owe it to yourself and your health to ask a number of simple questions:

- What are the side effects of this drug?
- What other drugs interact with this drug?
- Is there a better way to treat my medical condition than by subjecting myself to this drug?

SUMMARY

1. Americans and the medical establishment have a love affair with prescription medications.

2. Many of the drugs Americans take are unnecessary and are often prescribed to address the symptoms caused by other drugs.

3. Million-dollar advertising campaigns drive drug sales, normalizing the idea that pharmaceuticals can solve all our health problems.

4. Doctors are just as susceptible to sales pitches as their patients.

5. Pharmaceuticals are a billion-dollar business and the bottom line often takes precedence over concern for patients.

6. Antidepressant use has exploded even though the side effects can be severe, benefits minimal, and discontinuation difficult.

7. For more information, please visit www.hotzehwc.com/DrugDangers.

chapter
EIGHT

FIBROMYALGIA, CHRONIC FATIGUE SYNDROME, AND HYPOTHYROIDISM

JENNIFER'S STORY

After numerous office visits and prescription drugs, Jennifer's physician was exasperated and told her, "You will just have to live with this for the rest of your life."

Jennifer was young, beautiful, and vibrant, and had always led an active life. From grade school through college she had been actively involved in sports, drama, dance, and cheerleading, while maintaining her status as a top student. Her health and fitness were easily maintained and, as Jennifer realized later, much taken for granted.

After graduating from Boston College, Jennifer moved to Arizona where she became a paralegal. In her mid-30s, Jennifer noticed that her endurance level at the gym had begun to wane considerably. For someone who worked out daily and ran six days a week, this was unexpected and concerning. Sleep, something that

Jennifer never thought twice about before, suddenly became an issue. She tossed and turned and would wake up more worn out with each passing day. Despite feeling completely exhausted and fatigued, she was unable to get a restful night's sleep.

WORSENING SYMPTOMS

Over the next two years, Jennifer's symptoms slowly began to increase: insomnia, bone aching fatigue and muscle weakness, and then debilitating migraine headaches, excruciating menstrual cramps, and weight gain. Her entire body ached, from the joints in her hips to the muscles in her neck and shoulders. She was in constant pain. Jennifer also experienced recurring sinus infections, associated with a chronic sore throat and allergies. She was constantly sick.

Having been a very outgoing and social person, Jennifer now began to decline invitations to attend events or go on trips with friends. Her friends didn't understand what was going on and became angry, thinking that she no longer wanted to continue their relationship. She barely had enough energy to keep herself going, much less maintain relationships. She had nothing left to give at the end of the day.

To make matters worse, her health began to affect her job. By the time Jennifer arrived at the office each morning, she was already exhausted. She wondered how she would make it through the next eight hours. It took every ounce of energy just to concentrate and even more effort to physically stay at the office.

SEEKING HELP

Finally, Jennifer crashed. Her fatigue was so severe that she could hardly walk without becoming breathless. One day while sitting at her desk, hunched over, and shaking, feeling as if she were about to pass out, she realized that she could not keep going. She left her job that day and never returned. She was completely incapable of performing her job. Jennifer was only 37 years old, and her future looked bleak.

The next day, she visited the primary physician that she had been seeing since arriving in Phoenix. Jennifer planned out how she would once again relate all of her symptoms to him. Despite feeling worse than she had felt in her entire life, she was hoping beyond hope that he would listen to her intently, understand her predicament, and diagnose the underlying cause of her problem.

When the nurse roomed her in and asked her the reason for the visit, Jennifer told her of her problems. Immediately the nurse stated that she knew exactly what the matter was. "What a relief," Jennifer thought. When the doctor entered, he only allowed her to tell her story briefly. Without questioning her further, he pronounced that she was depressed. What? Jennifer had never mentioned anything about being depressed, not even once. Although she felt terrible, she knew she was not depressed.

The doctor handed her a sample case of Zoloft and sent her on her way with a pat on the back. He said, "This will make you feel better." She had been prescribed Xanax, antidepressants and sleep medications before, during previous doctor visits when she was attempting to solve her health problems. She hated how the drugs made her feel. They made her numb, as if she were viewing every-thing through a haze. The medications did help with her anxiety and sleep for a few days, but the effect was minimal and short-lived. Similar to a drug addict, she had to constantly increase the dose to get any effect. She didn't like feeling drugged and decided that she would not take the antidepressant.

TAKING A STEP BACK

Jennifer was left with no choice but to make the dreaded phone call to her parents in Texas. With fear of disappointment and no answer as to what was wrong with her, Jennifer told her parents that she was too sick to work. Her father immediately flew to Arizona to bring her home. She had to drop everything: leave her job, walk away from her friends, give up her independent life, give away her furniture, pack up what would fit into her SUV, and move back in with her parents. During the long, two-day drive back to Texas, Jennifer sat in the passenger seat, trembling and weak. She wondered how she had come to this place in her life.

In Texas, Jennifer's symptoms continued to worsen. She visited every kind of specialist imaginable. They ran blood test after blood test, all coming back with results in the "normal range." These specialists' offices were covered with walls of plaques and awards, yet their waiting rooms were filled with the sickest people she had ever seen. Nobody seemed well. Along the way, she collected diagnoses such as fibromyalgia, chronic fatigue syndrome, and irritable bowel syndrome (IBS) for which the doctors offered only antidepressants and antianxiety medications. She was told that she would just have to live with this for the rest of her life.

She was frightened. What if she were unable to keep a job? How would she support herself? She was young with her whole life ahead of her, but what kind of life would it be if she could barely get out of bed? Was this it? Would she have to suffer for the rest of her life?

ENCOURAGING PROGRESS

Upon visiting the Hotze Health & Wellness Center at the suggestion of family friends, Dr. Ellsworth explained that her problems were real and not in her head. The natural approach he recommended—using desiccated thyroid USP, replenishing and balancing the female hormones, treating adrenal fatigue, supplementing with vitamins and minerals, and starting on a yeast-free eating program—had almost immediate results.

Within several weeks after starting on the treatment program Jennifer began to regain her energy. Finally, she slept soundly, restfully. The migraine headaches, fatigue, insomnia, and menstrual difficulties all began to disappear. Eventually, and most importantly, she was able to return to work.

Looking back on her life, Jennifer says that she becomes livid thinking of how the doctors had treated her like a hypochondriac. She mourns the time that was wasted on misdiagnoses when hypothyroidism, so easily diagnosed, was her underlying problem all along. Now Jennifer is a passionate advocate for educating others about the far-reaching effects of hypothyroidism and the simple way to correct this condition.

FIBROMYALGIA, CHRONIC FATIGUE SYNDROME, AND IRRITABLE BOWEL SYNDROME

The CDC estimates that more than five million adults in the United States, nearly 2 percent of the population, have been diagnosed with or suffer from fibromyalgia. According to the National Fibromyalgia Association, there are between 15 and 20 million people who suffer with this syndrome. Whichever organization is correct, millions of people are plagued with this disorder. Studies also indicate that between one and four million Americans suffer from chronic fatigue syndrome, also known as chronic fatigue and immune dysfunction syndrome (CFIDS). These two syndromes are becoming increasingly more recognized in mainstream medicine.

Like Jennifer, these individuals suffer from debilitating fatigue, muscle weakness, joint pain, chronic headaches, tingling in the extremities, and insomnia. Fibromyalgia and chronic fatigue syndrome were not recognized as valid medical issues until the early 1990s. Prior to that, these patients were labeled as hypochondriacs because the symptoms of fibromyalgia and chronic fatigue fail to materialize in blood tests. Although both are considered clinical "diagnoses" today, current medicine has nothing to offer these patients beyond drugs to numb the pain. As in Jennifer's case, they are told that they will have to live with the pain and fatigue for the rest of their lives.

Mainstream medicine's attitude toward fibromyalgia and chronic fatigue is basically this: The patients are told that they are going to have to learn to deal with it and then are given pharmaceutical drugs to mask the symptoms and dull life along the way. Sufferers hold on to their diagnoses with clenched fists because it's the only answer they have. What good is a diagnosis without a solution? Mainstream medical sites for chronic fatigue and fibromyalgia offer support groups and outline the symptoms but have little to offer in the way of hope for healing. According to current medical thinking, the cause of fibromyalgia and chronic fatigue is mysterious and unknown.

Although both fibromyalgia and chronic fatigue syndrome are considered clinical "diagnoses" today, current medical thinking has nothing to offer patients beyond drugs to numb the pain.

ANOTHER MEDICAL MYSTERY?

By definition, neither fibromyalgia nor chronic fatigue syndrome is a diagnosis. A diagnosis is defined as the process of determining the nature and cause of a disease. Both of these disorders are syndromes for which today's medicine readily admits that it does not know the cause. The real question is this: What is the underlying cause or diagnosis of these two syndromes?

The primary cause of both these disorders is really quite straightforward. At the Hotze Health & Wellness Center, we have had great success treating the root cause of the symptoms of fibromyalgia and chronic fatigue. As we look closer at the symptoms of both these syndromes, you will recognize an uncanny resemblance to the underlying condition, which is the focus of this book: hypothyroidism.

—————— WORD WISE ——————

Fibromyalgia. This term is an amalgam of three Latin roots: *fibro* means "fibrous tissue," *myo* means "muscle," and *algia* means "pain."

DIAGNOSES OF MEDICALESE

Here's the scenario. You visit your doctor complaining of joint and muscle pain and hope to find out what's causing your symptoms. The doctor in his white coat nods as he listens to you describe how you are constantly tormented with pain in your joints and muscles, and with fatigue. He makes a few notes in your medical chart and then orders a battery of blood tests, X-rays, and CAT scans. On your return visit, your doctor proudly announces to you, "Well, I finally have the explanation for your problems." You breathe a sigh of relief. After a long pause, he finally gives you his diagnosis. "You have fibromyalgia."

"Wow! That sounds like something really ominous. At least I know that I have a real problem," you think.

But all your doctor did was translate your complaint into a Latin word describing joint and muscle pain and passed it off as a diagnosis. Do you recognize the circular thinking? Of course he can now charge you or your insurance company for giving you this diagnosis in Latin.

Your response should be, "Why do I have fibromyalgia? What is its cause?" I can assure you that he will not have an answer for you and will probably be offended that you had the gall to ask him this question in the first place. Many doctors do not like their ignorance to be exposed.

It's the same story with chronic fatigue syndrome. Although the pain and fatigue are very real and can often be debilitating, these two conditions are not actual diseases in and of themselves, but rather *symptoms* that have their roots in an underlying cause. Muscle pain and fatigue are very common symptoms of hypothyroidism. The solution for resolution of both of these disorders is to treat the most likely underlying cause of your symptoms, which is hypothyroidism. You would be amazed to see the dramatic results achieved in these conditions when they are treated with supplemental desiccated thyroid USP.

FIBROMYALGIA HISTORY

The American College of Rheumatology estimates that between six and 12 million people in the United States have fibromyalgia, 80 percent of whom are women.[77] This number splits the difference between the estimated number of people afflicted with this disorder by the CDC and National Fibromyalgia Association.

The symptoms of fibromyalgia have taken on a variety of names over the course of the last century. It has been called everything from muscular rheumatism to neurasthenia. Fibromyalgia has been thought to be a form of osteoarthritis or autoimmune disease.

Throughout the years one thing has remained constant, fibromyalgia is a controversial diagnosis.

The term *fibromyalgia* was coined in the late 1970s, but it wasn't until the 1990s that the American College of Rheumatology developed diagnostic criteria for fibromyalgia. An interesting note in the timeline of fibromyalgia's journey to mainstream medical acknowledgement is that the diagnosis received the official stamp of approval shortly on the heels of fibromyalgia drug trials that began in the late 1980s. Fibromyalgia awareness-marketing by pharmaceuticals began soon thereafter, along with the emergence of brand-new drugs to treat this "newly discovered" disease.

SYMPTOMS OF FIBROMYALGIA AND CHRONIC FATIGUE SYNDROME

The symptoms of fibromyalgia and chronic fatigue vary slightly. The differences lie in the "where" of the symptoms.

Individuals suffering from fibromyalgia chiefly complain of widespread pain, especially at certain tender points in the body, as well as debilitating fatigue. Chronic fatigue sufferers chiefly complain of extreme fatigue. Like Jennifer, a host of additional symptoms and diagnoses generally accompany fibromyalgia and chronic fatigue syndrome such as irritable bowel syndrome (IBS), depression, and anxiety.

According to the CDC, fibromyalgia is a disorder of unknown cause that is characterized by widespread pain, abnormal pain processing, sleep disturbance, fatigue, and often psychological distress. People with fibromyalgia may also have other symptoms, such as:

- morning stiffness

- tingling or numbness in hands and feet
- headaches, including migraines
- irritable bowel syndrome
- problems with thinking and memory (sometimes called "fibro fog")
- painful menstrual periods and other pain syndromes

The American College of Rheumatology (ACR) 2010 criteria is used for clinical diagnosis and severity classification of fibromyalgia.[78] The diagnosis is based on

- widespread pain index (WPI) ≥ 7 and a symptom severity scale (SS) ≥ 5 or WPI 3-6 and SS ≥ 9;
- Symptoms have been present at a similar level for at least three months;
- The patient does not have a disorder that would otherwise explain the pain.

DIAGNOSIS OF CHRONIC FATIGUE SYNDROME

The CDC criteria for establishing a diagnosis of chronic fatigue syndrome occurs if these three criteria are met:

1. The individual has severe chronic fatigue for six or more consecutive months that is not due to ongoing exertion or other medical conditions associated with fatigue (these other conditions need to be ruled out by a doctor after diagnostic tests have been conducted).
2. The fatigue significantly interferes with daily activities and work.
3. The individual concurrently has four or more of the following eight symptoms:

- postexertion malaise lasting more than 2 hours

- unrefreshing sleep
- significant impairment of short-term memory or concentration
- muscle pain
- multijoint pain without swelling or redness
- headaches of a new type, pattern, or severity
- tender cervical or axillary lymph nodes
- a sore throat that is frequent or recurring

SYMPTOM OVERLAP OF FIBROMYALGIA, CHRONIC FATIGUE SYNDROME, AND HYPOTHYROIDISM

The symptoms of fibromyalgia and chronic fatigue rarely travel alone. Most individuals experience a combination of many symptoms. As you can see, there is quite an overlap of symptoms between fibromyalgia, chronic fatigue, and hypothyroidism.

Symptoms	Fibromyalgia	CFS	Hypothyroidism
Joint pain and stiffness	X	X	X
Fatigue	X	X	X
Sleep disturbances	X	X	X
Headaches/migraines	X	X	X
Difficulty concentrating	X	X	X
Mental fog/"fibro fog"	X	X	X
Constipation/irritable bowel	X	X	X
Bloating	X	X	X
Painful menstrual periods	X		X
Dysmenorrhea	X		X
Depression	X	X	X
Panic attacks	X	X	X
Anxiety	X	X	X
Skin disorders (e.g., dry skin)	X		X
Muscle pain and weakness	X	X	X

Nausea	X	X	X
Dizziness	X	X	X
Sore throat	X	X	X
Tingling or numbness in extremities	X		X
Cold extremities	X		X
Memory loss	X	X	X
Shortness of breath	X	X	X
Increased allergy symptoms	X	X	X
Heightened chemical sensitivity	X	X	X
Blurred vision	X	X	X
Sensitivity to light	X	X	X
Weight loss or gain	X	X	X
Chest pain	X	X	X
Chills and night sweats		X	X
Chronic cough		X	X

FIBROMYALGIA DRUGS

Pharmaceutical drug trials for fibromyalgia began in the late 1980s, and by the time that mainstream medicine deemed fibromyalgia a real disease, the drug companies were poised and ready to unveil their marketing plan.

This was hardly a coincidence. Drug companies dream up syndromes and so-called "diseases" so that they can sell drugs. The pharmaceutical companies then conduct their own studies and manipulate the data to demonstrate that their drug is really safer than a placebo in treating the new disorder that they have concocted.

As we saw in Chapter 7, the so-called "scientific" articles for publication in medical journals are created by writers at public relations firms. Respected academic medical doctors are paid to lend their name to the article for publication. These academicians are then paid fees to lecture on the benefits of the drug at medical conferences.

Lyrica, originally a drug for epileptic seizures made by Pfizer, was approved by the FDA in 2007 for the treatment of fibromyalgia. Eli Lilly was quick on Pfizer's heels in getting its antidepressant, Cymbalta, approved for treatment of fibromyalgia one year later. Now the pharmaceutical companies had the drugs for the treatment of fibromyalgia. The only thing left to do was to create a need for these drugs within the American public. Only in the pharmaceutical industry are the laws of supply and demand reversed. Before selling the drug, you must first sell the disease that creates demand for the drug.

PROMOTING A DISEASE

Pfizer and Eli Lilly effectively assisted the American public in understanding this new disorder. The marketing of fibromyalgia was disguised as a campaign for fibromyalgia awareness.[79] Eli Lilly and

Pfizer donated more than $6 million to nonprofit groups for medical conferences and educational campaigns in the first three quarters of 2008. The drug makers spent more on fibromyalgia awareness than they had on Alzheimer's and diabetes awareness, falling just short of the money spent on cancer, AIDS, and depression awareness. Pfizer and Lilly spent a whopping $125 million and $128.4 million respectively on advertising their fibromyalgia drugs in 2008.

Marketing fibromyalgia to the public paid off. The sales of these drugs have been phenomenal for both companies. Lilly's Cymbalta sales skyrocketed from $442 million in 2007 to $3.2 billion in 2011, while Pfizer's Lyrica followed suit, increasing sales from $395 million in 2007 to $3.4 billion in 2011.

These drugs are touted to reduce fibromyalgia pain, although the results are marginal at best. The side effects of both drugs include nausea, dizziness, weight gain, constipation, blurry vision, trouble concentrating, drowsiness, swelling of the hands and feet, feeling "high," and suicidal thoughts. Ironically, some of these side effects are already symptoms of fibromyalgia. Many fibromyalgia patients are simultaneously taking both Lyrica and Cymbalta.

DRUGS TO MASK SYMPTOMS

The sufferers of fibromyalgia and CFS have become easy targets for the drug industry. Those complaining of fibromyalgia and chronic fatigue are left with treatments that are only meant to mask their symptoms. The root cause of their symptoms, hypothyroidism, goes unrecognized and is left untreated, resulting in additional symptoms and, as always, more drugs. Symptom after symptom is treated with pharmaceutical drugs or surgery. Joint and muscle pain? Take an anti-inflammatory. Depressed? Take an antidepressant. Anxious? Here's an antianxiety drug. Menstrual problems? Try birth control pills. Chronic menstrual problems? It's probably time for a hysterectomy. And the story goes on and on. The symptoms and drugs begin to multiply. Unfortunately, there is never a happy ending for those who stay on the drug merry-go-round.

Hypothyroidism can cause a host of health problems including all the symptoms found in fibromyalgia and chronic fatigue syndrome. Medical doctors have told us that these conditions have unknown causes. Sometimes the illusion of knowledge is the greatest impediment to solving problems. Over the last 120 years, millions of patients have been successfully treated with desiccated thyroid for the very symptoms found in these two syndromes.

In Jennifer's case, replenishing her thyroid using desiccated thyroid USP, enabled her to get her life back. What about your life?

SUMMARY

1. Fibromyalgia and chronic fatigue syndrome are controversial diagnoses that have nevertheless become increasingly common in recent years.
2. Although the medical establishment considers the cause of fibromyalgia and CFS mysterious, their symptoms significantly overlap with those of hypothyroidism.
3. The pharmaceutical industry has come up with drugs that mask the symptoms of both conditions but do not address their underlying cause.
4. Big Pharma has heavily promoted both the medications and the conditions they claim to treat.
5. For more information, please visit www.hotzehwc.com/FibromyalgiaSymptoms.

WOMEN'S HEALTH AND HYPOTHYROIDISM

I t was never my intention to develop my medical practice around the treatment of women's female hormone problems. Although we treat men, 80 percent of our guests are women.

My initial plan for my medical career was to become a surgeon and, in fact, I completed one year of a surgical residency at St. Joseph's Hospital in Houston, Texas. At this time, Janie and I had four children, and I decided that I had to make a living, so I entered the field of emergency medicine in 1977 for five years and then transitioned to family medicine in Houston. Subsequently, I entered the field of allergy medicine in 1989 and opened a small medical practice with one staff member in Katy, Texas, a suburb just west of Houston. This was the genesis of what has become the Hotze Health & Wellness Center with two allied enterprises, Physician's Preference Vitamin Store and Hotze Pharmacy, a compounding pharmacy that specializes solely in preparing bioidentical hormones and carries only two pharmaceutical drugs, fluconazole to treat yeast, and Armour Thyroid. These enterprises now have more than 90 team members who are "A" players and who have been recruited to provide extraordinary hospitality and Ritz-Carlton service to our guests.

During my first three years of practice, I treated patients for both airborne and food allergy disorders in combination with vitamin supplementation, and I also treated patients for overgrowth of yeast in the intestines. In 1992 Dr. Richard Mabray, an obstetrician and gynecologist who also treated patients for allergic disorders, introduced me to the concept of checking and treating my patients for hypothyroidism, specifically for autoimmune thyroiditis. His recommended use of desiccated thyroid USP for patients, when indicated, made a significant difference in the health and well-being of my allergy patients. Yet, there were still other patients who had some improvement but who continued to have symptoms related to female hormonal imbalance.

PATTERNS IN WOMEN

As I noted earlier, I began to recognize an interesting pattern among my allergy patients. While my male patients typically had a lifelong history of allergies, many women were seeking my care for assistance with allergy problems that had appeared, seemingly out of the blue, in midlife. They were complaining of recurrent sinus infections, bronchitis, asthma, skin disorders, and food allergies. For some women, childbirth seemed to trigger their allergies. For others, the onset of allergies was associated with a change in their menstrual cycles, or after a hysterectomy, or at menopause.

It became obvious to me that there was a relationship between allergic disorders and female hormone fluctuations in midlife. However, I was an allergist, not a gynecologist. When I determined that a woman needed help with hormonal problems, I referred her to a gynecologist.

Then, one day after work, in February 1996, I was sitting at my desk, going through my mail, when I came across a monograph by

Julian Whitaker, MD, on the therapeutic use of natural hormones. Because I was having great success treating hypothyroidism with natural thyroid replacement, I was eager to read what Dr. Whitaker had to say about this topic.

That evening at home, I read the chapter on natural thyroid. Dr. Whitaker's writings confirmed my own experience in treating patients with hypothyroidism. Whitaker wrote that symptoms, not blood tests, were the best way to diagnose and manage hypothyroidism and that the use of a natural desiccated thyroid extract, such as Armour Thyroid, was the best way to treat this very common, yet often unrecognized, condition.

Dr. Whitaker's monograph contained chapters on other hormones, including estrogen, progesterone, testosterone, dehydro-epiandrosterone (DHEA), pregnenolone and growth hormone. I read them all. Until then, the concept of using bioidentical hormones for the treatment of women's hormone problems, was completely foreign to me.

By the end of the evening, I understood the therapeutic potential of bioidentical hormones. It was a concept that I had never been taught in medical school. Now I realized the difference between natural bioidentical hormones and the counterfeit hormones produced by drug companies.

LEARNING FROM OTHERS

There is an old adage that states, "When the student is ready, the teacher will appear." I was that eager student. The day after I read Dr. Whitaker's monograph, I walked into guest room 2 at my center, and there, sitting on the examination table, was Larke, a long-time patient of mine in her late 30s. She held out an audio cassette and said, "Dr. Hotze, would you like to learn about natural progesterone therapy? This is a tape by Dr. John Lee."

"That's interesting," I replied. "I just spent last night reading about natural progesterone and would be very interested in listening to what this doctor has to say about its use."

On my 30-minute drive home that evening, I listened to the tape. Dr. Lee had been recommending natural progesterone supplementation to his female patients for almost 20 years with amazing results. On his audiotape, he explained how premenstrual complaints, reproductive difficulties, and menopausal symptoms could be triggered by the inevitable decline in a woman's production of progesterone, which usually began in her mid-thirties.

Dr. Lee's descriptions of his patients' symptoms were the same symptoms of which my patients were complaining.

"Natural progesterone could be the missing link that could help these women," I thought.

The next day, I reached Dr. Lee, who practiced in California, by phone and asked him, "Where in the world do I get natural progesterone?" Dr. Lee replied that progesterone could be purchased with a prescription through a compounding pharmacy. A few days later, a local compounding pharmacist, Phil Pylant, dropped by my office to introduce himself and offer his services. It turned out that Phil was a highly respected compounding pharmacist who taught other pharmacists how to compound prescriptions. Phil told me that he was not only familiar with natural female hormones, but that he could compound natural progesterone and the natural human estrogens (estradiol, estrone, and estriol) for my patients.

Here I was, the eager student who wanted to learn how to help my patients get better, and within three (3) days three (3) different teachers had arrived: Dr. Whitaker, my patient Larke, and Dr. Lee.

That has been the story of my life. "Ask and you shall be given. Seek and you shall find" (Matthew. 7:7).

THYROID AND FERTILITY

Progesterone is essential in balancing a woman's estrogen hormones, and works very well in correcting estrogen dominance in women. In so doing, progesterone enhances thyroid function at the cellular level. As you read in Chapter 4, hypothyroidism in women is often a consequence of estrogen dominance. Some of the most serious complications of estrogen dominance include breast cancer, infertility issues, and miscarriages. While not indicated in every case, when it is, desiccated thyroid hormone supplementation can mean the difference between "Guess what, honey. We're pregnant!" and "I just don't understand why I can't get pregnant."

The average success rate of infertility clinics is 25 percent. That means that infertility clinics have a 75 percent failure rate. What's underappreciated is that proper assimilation of thyroid hormones into the cells is essential in order to conceive and to maintain a pregnancy. It has been gratifying to see just how many women who have suffered unsuccessfully through traditional infertility treatments, have experienced the joy of motherhood after being evaluated and treated by the physicians at our center.

A LOCAL JUDGE'S STORY

A prominent local judge came in for her annual follow-up evaluation, and when she saw me in the front office area, she exclaimed with glee for everyone to hear, "Dr. Hotze, I have been telling everyone how you got me pregnant!" Needless to say, that stopped me in my tracks. I had visions of headlines in the *Houston Chronicle* reading, "Dr. Hotze Gets Local Judge Pregnant," and I cringed at the thought. Her remarks elicited an immediate response from me. "Wait a minute now, Judge. I didn't get you pregnant. Your husband did. I simply helped balance your hormones in order to give you the best chance to get pregnant." She went on to explain that she had recently given birth to her first baby and how elated she felt. She had seen infertility specialists without success and had given up on the hope of ever having a baby. Her pregnancy was a welcome surprise, and she was shouting my praises from the rooftops. She attributed it to the treatment recommendations I had made, primarily thyroid hormone supplementation. I just wished that she had worded it differently when she complimented me to her friends and associates!

The most common cause of infertility and miscarriages is hormonal deficiency and imbalance. This includes the thyroid, sex, and adrenal hormones. Remember, they work together synergistically, and when properly balanced, enhance one another's functions and actions.

Although we are not an infertility clinic, some of our guests, who balanced their hormones and conceived, have characterized us as a fertility clinic. When a woman's hormones are present in healthy amounts and in balance, she has a much better chance to conceive.

IN HER OWN WORDS: ELIZABETH'S STORY

Today I am a renewed person. I say this because I am now the happy, healthy, and active person I used to be before my problems with autoimmune thyroiditis, yeast infections, and deficient progesterone levels began, not to mention the inability of numerous doctors to fix these problems.

I had always had trouble with hormones, even in my early twenties, but finding a doctor to correct that problem was impossible because all they wanted to do was put me on birth control pills. I had always had an adverse reaction to any birth control pills that I took. As long as I had no stress in my life, enough sleep, and I was not ill, my hormone levels were fine, but the minute I encountered stress or an illness, became more active, or did not get much sleep a few nights in a row, it would throw my hormone levels off. My husband and I had been trying, and I mean we tried hard, to have another child for over ten years with no success.

How It Began

Before all of my symptoms began, I woke up at 4:15 a.m. almost every day to work out, but then I began feeling like I was being drugged or that I was drunk all of the time. I began having digestive problems and severe acid reflux. I found it very hard to stay awake during my hour trip to work during the week, even after what I thought was a good night's sleep. I was late for work every day because I could hardly drag myself out of bed. After being an early morning person for many years, it was real hard for me to be able to arise early in the morning. I would come home from work, eat, and go to bed. My family and my boss began to worry about me because I was just not the same person who had previously awakened early and had kept going all day long. Sex was completely out of the question because, let's face it, I did not have the energy to participate in physical activity at the time. All I wanted to do was sleep.

I came to my wit's end when, for no apparent reason, I gained 20 pounds in two months and could barely think or walk in a straight line. Functioning physically was a huge chore for me during that time. I sought help from 11 doctors in various medical fields. Several of them said I had no thyroid or hormone problems, and several wanted to put me on antidepressants. One even suggested that I seek psychiatric help for my condition. I am ashamed to say that I wanted to slap that one. Then I came across an article that Dr. Hotze had written and realized that the symptoms of the patient that he referenced in that article were exactly the same symptoms that I was having.

Changing Direction

I saw Dr. Hotze in the latter part of May. He put me on hormone replacement therapy, thyroid medication, and various other medications, vitamins, minerals, and supplements. I was instructed to go on a diet free from yeast and sugar. This is what I had previously considered the 'fun stuff' to eat. Even though I thought he was out of his mind, I did everything that I was instructed to do. At the time, I did not understand how his program could work. I waited until the beginning of June to begin the eating plan, so I had time to purchase the things needed for the diet and, admittedly, to psyche myself up for it.

Four months later, I had lost a little over 20 pounds but, more importantly, I had the energy, vitality and libido that I had before all of my problems began. That is not all, because there was icing on the cake. I finally got pregnant after trying for over 10 years! When I was about six months pregnant, I was still asking my doctor if he was sure I was pregnant because I still could not believe it. My youngest son will be five in July and has brought so much joy to my life. I could not imagine my life without him.

AUTOIMMUNE THYROIDITIS AND PREGNANCY

Much has already been said about the intricate connection that thyroid has with the other hormonal systems within the human body. Yet, we must once again explore together a less than obvious connection: thyroid and pregnancy. Most women have never considered that thyroid issues might be the cause of their difficulties in conceiving a baby and carrying it to term. Yet, it is increasingly common. During pregnancy, a woman's body requires approximately 50 percent more thyroid production in order to support the baby's growth and development.[80] Thus, if a woman is not producing or utilizing enough thyroid hormone, a miscarriage may result. Autoimmune thyroiditis is a further complication.

In a previous chapter, we discussed autoimmune thyroiditis, the condition that results when the immune system makes thyroid antibodies, which attack the thyroid gland. In 2009 Dr. Alex Stagnaro–Green, a professor of medicine, obstetrics, and gynecology at Touro University College of Medicine in Hackensack, NJ, described the impact of thyroid conditions on pregnancy.[81] This study sought to determine the incidence of autoimmune thyroiditis during and immediately after pregnancy. The results revealed that the incidence of miscarriages in women with autoimmune thyroiditis, but with normal thyroid hormone blood tests, was 50 percent higher than women in the study who had no antibodies to their thyroid. Sixteen percent of the women with thyroid antibodies miscarried.[82] Another complication that arises in women with autoimmune thyroiditis is premature delivery.

Even when there are normal thyroid hormone levels in the blood, autoimmune thyroiditis adversely affects the cells' ability to properly utilize thyroid hormones. This leads to a hypothyroid condition within the cells. In a study done in Italy in 2006,[83] researchers demonstrated that women with thyroid antibodies who were given supplemental thyroid hormone during the early stages of their pregnancy, miscarried four times less than women with the same condition who were given a placebo. Clearly, thyroid hormone replacement enhances the ability of women with autoimmune thyroiditis to maintain a healthy pregnancy and deliver a full-term baby. Every pregnant woman should be tested for the presence of thyroid antibodies. Unfortunately this is rarely done.

If your health began to gradually decline after the birth of your child, you are not alone. The extreme fatigue, recurrent infections, "baby blues," inability to lose weight, and menstrual irregularities are a shared experience for many women. Rather than masking these symptoms with pharmaceutical drugs, such as sleep medication or antidepressants, the underlying cause should be addressed. Since estrogen dominance is often the first hormonal domino that begins the cascade of symptoms, this is where we will begin.

PROGESTERONE DEFICIENCY/ESTROGEN DOMINANCE AFTER DELIVERY

The hormonal imbalance that develops after childbirth is primarily due to the precipitous drop in progesterone, which leads to estrogen dominance. Progesterone is the key hormone of pregnancy. Progesterone promotes gestation, namely, pregnancy, hence its name. During pregnancy, the placenta, which belongs to the baby, produces progesterone at levels significantly higher than the levels a woman's ovaries normally produce. After the birth of the baby, the placenta is expelled, resulting in a steep decline in the progesterone level. The ovaries, which have been switched off during the last half of the pregnancy, must now turn on and begin producing the female hormones. If the ovaries are sluggish, not producing adequate hormones, problems ensue. This is a common cause of the typical "baby blues" experienced by many women. Progesterone is known for its mood-elevating effects.

When a woman's postdelivery progesterone levels are in the tank, her estrogen levels remain high. This results in estrogen becoming the dominant hormone. Estrogen dominance reveals itself premenstrually with symptoms such as breast tenderness, fluid retention, weight gain, headaches, severe menstrual cramps, irregular and heavy periods, and mood-related symptoms such as anxiety, panic attacks, or depression. Estrogen dominance also becomes a catalyst for many other hormone issues.

Estrogen dominance causes the liver to produce increasing levels of TBG, which binds thyroid hormones, making them less receptive to the cells. When thyroid hormones are bound in the blood by TBG, they are no longer available to enter the cells to create energy. At a time when a woman needs to feel superhuman to provide nurturing care to her infant, she feels overwhelmed instead.

My five daughters have given birth to 12 children to date. I instructed each one of them to start taking bioidentical progesterone the morning following their delivery. They all did and felt exceptionally well after delivery, never experiencing any problems with fatigue and depression.

ADRENAL FATIGUE IN WOMEN

In the same way that hypothyroidism can develop after giving birth, estrogen dominance also plays a role in postpartum adrenal fatigue. The higher-than-normal ratio of estrogen to progesterone that can develop after childbirth also causes an increase in levels of cortisol-binding globulin, which binds cortisol in the blood. Cortisol is the hormone that the adrenal gland produces to deal with chronic stress. With elevated levels of cortisol-binding hormone, there is less free cortisol available to enter the cell membranes and activate receptors inside the cell.

In addition, estrogen dominance interferes with the release of cortisol from the adrenal cortex.

Cortisol is made from progesterone. When progesterone levels dramatically decline after pregnancy, so does cortisol production. So whether it is an inhibited output of cortisol from the adrenal cortex, leading to a decrease in cortisol production, or whether cortisol is bound in the bloodstream by cortisol-binding globulin, both conditions result in adrenal fatigue.

As you age, your adrenal glands produce less cortisol. This inevitably leads to adrenal fatigue to one degree or another.

STEPS GOING FORWARD

If you have given birth and are experiencing the symptoms of hypothyroidism or adrenal fatigue, you should find a doctor who is experienced in dealing with these issues and will offer you natural solutions to correct them. The treatment of postpartum blues is very simple; you just need to be provided with adequate amounts of progesterone and desiccated thyroid hormone.

Postpartum thyroid issues are sometimes temporary, but one-third of all women who are diagnosed with the condition will continue to experience problems. Those women who find it a temporary condition are more likely to succumb to it in future pregnancies.

Women who are fortunate enough to find a physician to evaluate them properly during and after their pregnancies for postpartum thyroiditis and hypothyroidism will usually be prescribed Synthroid, or its equivalent, as the preferred method of treatment. If this happens to you, be sure to ask your physician to prescribe desiccated thyroid, which contains both the active T3 thyroid molecule and the inactive T4 molecule. This is because your body may have trouble converting the T4 thyroid molecule to the active T3 molecule. To get optimal results from your thyroid medication, your body needs to receive what it requires most: active T3 hormone.

In my practice, we rarely prescribe the synthetic T4 versions of thyroid medication alone. There is an occasional patient who can only tolerate low doses of T3 or no T3 at all. In these individuals we have to make special adjustments to the ratio of T4 to T3 by using specially compounded preparations of our thyroid supplements to address their needs.

SUMMARY

1. Estrogen dominance can lead to hypothyroidism, which also affects fertility, making conception more difficult.
2. Pregnancy exacerbates hormonal imbalances that can lead to hypothyroidism.
3. Pregnancy can increase the likelihood of progesterone deficiency, estrogen dominance, and adrenal fatigue.
4. Hypothyroidism can explain why many women suffer from post-partum symptoms.
5. For more information, please visit www.hotzehwc.com/HowChildbirthAffectsHormones.

chapter
TEN

TREATMENT OF HYPOTHYROIDISM

ROBERTO'S STORY

R oberto learned English by diligently listening to talk radio every day. It was this same ambitious drive and resolve that brought him to the United States from Venezuela in 1996 when he began working in the oil and gas industry. Throughout his fast-paced career, Roberto continued to listen to the radio and refine his skills in understanding the English language. Roberto had been a *Health & Wellness Solutions* listener for more than ten years before the message began to hit home.

PREMATURELY SLOWING DOWN

At 46 years old, Roberto was exhausted. He had always been active in the gym and sports with a particular love for Tae Kwan Do, but his strength and endurance were slipping. Upon a visit to his physician for a routine physical, Roberto was placed on Lipitor to treat his high cholesterol. After starting the medication, he was asked to come into the physician's office for continuous blood work.

Coming from a family full of physicians, Roberto had great confidence in the medical community, but things just weren't adding up. Why all the blood work? After a few months, he finally asked why he was constantly being tested. The physician told him that the cholesterol-lowering drug was causing problems with his liver. It seemed like common sense to Roberto that he should get off the drug because the risks outweighed the benefit. Roberto's physical stamina had been in a downward slide for the previous five years and the cholesterol problem finally led him to take an assessment of his health.

Roberto was so exhausted that it was all he could do to get through work and still have enough energy to play an active role in the lives of his wife and two daughters. The trips to the gym and Tae Kwan Do had long been discontinued due to severe muscle pain. Exhausted from the day, he would fall into bed only to find a sleepless night ahead of him. He had so many things he wanted to do, but his body just wouldn't cooperate.

During a trip to visit his father in Venezuela, they had a conversation that was a wake-up call for Roberto. He was extremely fatigued while working with his father on the family's farm. When his father noticed Roberto's condition, he turned to him and said, "Roberto, how can you be tired? I'm your *father*. I'm much older than you, yet I'm not tired. How can *you* be tired?" Roberto knew that his father was right. Instead of feeling he was in his prime, Roberto felt he was an old man. He realized that he needed to take action to regain his health. He remembered my radio program, to which he had been faithfully listening for more than ten years, and how it discussed solutions to the same problems he was having. Roberto decided it was time to take charge of his health, so he called my center to set up an appointment.

RECOVERED STAMINA

Based upon his clinical presentation, Roberto's physician at the center, Dr. Don Ellsworth, recommended that he begin a regimen that included natural desiccated thyroid, bioidentical testosterone, and vitamin and mineral supplementation. Roberto also adopted the yeast-free eating program, which resulted in his losing 30 pounds. Within six months, his energy had significantly improved. After a year on the program Roberto felt fantastic. He was back in the gym lifting weights and was once again involved in Tae Kwan Do. Physically and mentally, in every aspect—decision making, processing data, concentration, and physical stamina—Roberto is now at the top of his game. What a difference it has made in his marriage and family life! His dedication and commitment to health is an example to all of us. By partnering with a team of health professionals who gave him the right tools and support, Roberto was able to restore his health and get his life back.

Roberto suffered from classic symptoms of hypothyroidism, complicated by hormonal decline. He had suffered from insomnia, brain fog, extreme fatigue, and muscle aches and weakness. His cholesterol was elevated, another classic sign of hypothyroidism. Had it been a female who had presented to her physician, complaining of these symptoms, she probably would have been diagnosed with fibromyalgia or chronic fatigue syndrome and given a prescription for an antidepressant. Instead, Roberto had been given a prescription for Lipitor, an anticholesterol statin drug, by his previous physician, and sent on his way. Regardless of gender, medicine's solution is always the same: drugs, drugs, and more drugs to mask the symptoms rather than addressing the underlying problem.

THE HOTZE APPROACH TO TREATMENT

Like Roberto, the people who come to see us at the Hotze Health & Wellness Center routinely have seen a host of other physicians and been placed on a variety of medications, most of them psychiatric drugs of some sort. I'd say 75 percent of the women we see are either currently taking, have taken, or were prescribed but didn't take some kind of psychiatric preparation, antidepressant, antianxiety medication, or worse.

They just never got better, so they turn to us oftentimes as a last resort. I can't tell you the number of people who said, "I've heard you can help. If you can't help me, I don't know where I can turn." Patients aren't just after symptom relief; they want to get their lives back.

We see this in women when they hit their 40s and their hormones go south. They can't keep up the pace, and they've got a couple of kids. They can't function, don't feel well, can't sleep, and can't think. Their romantic moods and inclinations are gone. They're tired. They've got headaches. They're sick. All they want to do is go home and crawl into bed. They're moody, grouchy, agitated, angry— and their relationships with loved ones have often soured. They're not the people they used to be, and they feel bad about that.

We partner with them to restore their health so that once their health is restored, their lives can be transformed. If their lives are transformed, their world is improved, and this is done naturally.

LISTENING TO EVERY GUEST

When guests first call, a guest consultant explains our program. From the very first moment, we listen. An initial question might be, "What's going on in your life?" We share what we offer and see if there's a match. If there is, the prospective guest goes through an extensive questionnaire online. A questionnaire specialist goes over that questionnaire to make sure everything is right. He goes through a very extensive medical history, family history, past medical history, chief complaint, and any current medications guests are on. All this information is gathered on electronic medical records.

The first visit is always in the morning. Guests come to the center and are evaluated: Their blood is drawn. We do electrocardiogram and bone density tests. For women, we do breast thermograms. A physician or someone from the medical team then comes in and visits with the guest for approximately an hour, covering all his or her history, asking questions and listening. This may be the most important part of the treatment—not discounting what guests have to say but hearing their stories.

Each guest can interact with the physician, the physician's assistant, or nurse practitioner, and develop a transformative conversation where a series of questions are asked by both parties to try to determine the best course of action and lay out a plan that will help put the guest on a path of health and wellness.

PARTNERS FOR GOOD HEALTH

The people on our medical team are like coaches, and our guests are like health athletes: We're trying to get them into the health Olympics and want them to win a gold medal. We can give them the regimen, oversee it, help them train, and give counsel and advice. But ultimately, they have to embrace the program, and the accomplishments are theirs.

The goal of our transformative conversation is to build a relationship because when our guests come in, they're often confused about their state of health. They feel isolated because they don't know what's going on. They're isolated from not only their doctor but their family, and their friends, and even themselves. They've pulled back into a cocoon, are feeling poorly, and don't know what to do or who to turn to.

As my mentor, Dan Sullivan, has taught me, what we want to provide for them is leadership. We want to provide them with direction so they have clarity in their thinking—show them and explain to them why they feel the way they feel. Developing a relationship enables them to have confidence because they have somebody they can trust who will not only provide leadership on their journey but also stay with them and help put them on a path of health and wellness naturally, without the use of pharmaceutical drugs. By giving them creative ideas, we help them achieve new capabilities so they're no longer powerless.

The people on our medical team are like coaches and our guests are like health athletes: We're trying to get them into the health Olympics and want them to win a gold medal.

ALLEVIATING FEARS

What we do, then, by establishing clarity in their thinking, confidence because of the relationships, and new capabilities because of the creative ideas we give them, is help guests eliminate the dangers that they're fearful of. Guests come in thinking, "If I feel like this now, will I be alive in five or ten years?"

What are they concerned about? They hear all about high blood pressure problems, strokes, diabetes, heart disease, cancer, degenerative arthritis, Alzheimer's disease, depression—all these things that are talked about and advertised on television. They feel as if they're going to fall into a black hole of medical problems. By getting them on the path to health and wellness so they have clarity in their thinking and confidence in new capabilities, we can eliminate their fear.

By limiting their perceived dangers, we help them capture the opportunities in their lives so they can take advantage of them and maximize their strengths. We not only want to help them become healthy; we want to help them improve their lives.

ONGOING RELATIONSHIPS

We have ongoing programs in which we're constantly in contact with our guests. During the initial visit, they're here four hours, and they get a program with a printout and a binder of what they're going to do. Our professionals counsel them on vitamins, the importance of vitamins, and what we've recommended for them. They also consult with the on-site pharmacist about their bioidentical hormones.

After that, guests can always be in contact with us through our phone nurse department. They can call the phone nurse any time from Monday through Friday during the day for counseling on any problem or aspect of their treatment regimen, whether it involves allergies, food, yeast treatment, hormones, or vitamins, minerals, and nutrients. Our professionals can help guide guests on making adjustments in their treatment regimen immediately so they don't have to wait a week for a doctor to call them back if the doctor gets stacked up.

We get hundreds of calls every day from our guests who have questions. We also keep in communication daily through e-mail or by putting information on our blog and website, communicating ideas about health and what we can do to keep guests on a path to health and wellness. This is important because treatment often means changing some habits or patterns of living and eating, and sometimes that's difficult for people.

AN EXTENDED COMMUNITY

We also host conferences based on the relationships we've built with guests who are so enthusiastic that we call them ambassadors. They may go on television or radio programs with us, such as my radio show from noon to 1 p.m. central time, Monday through Thursday, on top-rated KSEV talk radio in Houston. Our guests' success stories encourage other people in the community. Guests also write their stories, host home parties for us in the area, and participate in symposiums.

In the symposiums, we also help guests in their own personal and business lives to adopt principles that help them be more successful. We want their health success to translate into success in everything they do.

There's additional information, and courses are available as well: We're launching an online university called Hotze University that will enable our guests to study various health concepts online in short vignettes, covering topics ranging from what kind of thyroid hormones to take to symptoms of hypothyroidism, historical background, sex hormones, adrenal hormones, eating programs, and vitamins.

Our education initiatives also include learning from the work of success gurus and others who emphasize having a positive mental attitude. On our staff we read a book a month by experts, inspirational authors such as Zig Ziglar, John Maxwell, and Jim Collins, and have done so for more than ten years—information that is also imparted to our guests.

ENVIRONMENT MATTERS

On top of all this, when guests enter this transformative relationship, we offer a hospitality environment. When you come to our center, there's nobody in a white coat, scrubs, or tennis shoes. Everybody's in a nice black suit. You walk in, and it feels as if you're coming to a very nice hotel like the Ritz. In fact, we've studied the philosophy of the Ritz and have had their people train our people.

Why is that important to health? We want to create an environment that both cultivates a sense of well-being and fulfills even the unexpressed wishes and needs of our guests. We want guests to feel they're prized and honored people. If you've ever stayed at a Ritz and compared it to a Motel 6 or Holiday Inn, you know what I'm talking about. They treat you nicely. They smile. They remember your name. They're always there to serve you. They make you feel special. It's the same way at our center. When people come, they feel very special— as opposed to most doctors' offices, where you feel you're intruding on their time. The medical profession on the whole has no concept of guest service or customer service. It's not taught or exemplified, and an ungracious attitude permeates the clinical world.

MY LARGER VISION OF MEDICINE

I'm a free enterprise capitalist and do not believe in socialism, but if I were the surgeon general and had the power to mandate, I would mandate that every doctor learn about hypothyroidism and start treating guests, or patients, when indicated, with desiccated thyroid extract and see how they do.

I'd also like to see doctors think more broadly about endocrine problems. All the hormones are interactive, particularly the sex hormones and the adrenal hormones. When we treat, we treat for all three classes of hormones: the sex hormones, the adrenal hormones, and the thyroid hormones because they work together synergistically. Doctors need to think in terms of hormonal deficiencies and declines as causing a majority of the health problems in midlife that can lead to a host of degenerative conditions as people mature.

I'd encourage doctors to rely less on pharmaceutical drugs instead of having a country that makes up 5 percent of the world's population yet uses 42 percent of the world's drugs at enormous cost to our health care system and general well-being.

I'd encourage education on natural approaches to health including hormonal declines and imbalances, bioidentical hormones, and nutritional training. And I'd encourage a movement toward treating empirically, using therapeutic trials of desiccated thyroid, titrating doses to see if people's symptoms improve.

And I'd train doctors to question. Always ask why. Never believe anything just because somebody says it's so. Why is it so? What's the cause? Why should we use a drug? Questioning is how I arrived at the eight-point treatment regimen I describe in Chapter 1. I started with allergies and vitamins and then treated for yeast because many allergy patients get infections, use antibiotics, and then get yeast problems that cause a host of other problems. So I'd treat them for that. If they still didn't get well, I'd keep asking questions. I found out about thyroid and when thyroid didn't work on everybody, I found out about sex hormones. Then I found out about adrenal hormones. Then I found out about a good eating program. It took me ten years of continually asking questions to get my eight-point treatment regimen to where it is now. And I continue to ask questions every day.

What follows are some of the specific elements of treatment and attitudes toward care that so often prove helpful for our guests.

QUESTIONING THE VALUE OF THYROID TESTS

Since 1973 medical doctors have considered the thyroid-stimulating hormone (TSH) blood test to be the "gold standard" for detecting hypothyroidism.[84] As we saw in Chapter 2, the TSH is not a thyroid hormone. Instead, it's a hormone secreted by the pituitary gland in the brain to stimulate the thyroid gland to produce thyroid hormone. The pituitary gland regulates the thyroid gland's hormone production. Think of the thyroid gland as a race horse and the pituitary gland as the jockey. The TSH is the whip that the jockey uses on the horse when it is running too slow.

When the TSH level is elevated, this indicates that the thyroid gland is not producing enough thyroid hormone and that thyroid hormone supplementation is needed. The accepted reference range for TSH is critical. But as we covered in detail in Chapter 3, what's considered the "normal" range for TSH is excessively broad. What's more, lab results can vary widely and are therefore unreliable.

It seems unwise for a physician to rely solely on TSH when his patient's history, symptoms, and physical examination clearly indicate a hypothyroid condition. In this case, the prudent treatment would be to offer a clinical trial of thyroid hormone supplementation.

Thousands of men and women are left untreated because the TSH misses the mark. Relying on the TSH alone has led physicians to treat the lab value rather than the patient. It is assumed that the hypothalamus and pituitary are functioning properly without being affected by aging, toxins, or defects. The TSH blood test also presumes that every bit of thyroid hormone that is in your blood is utilized in your cells. We have demonstrated how this is not the case.

Unfortunately, there is no blood test that indicates how much active thyroid we have in our cells. Several conditions that we have already described, such as autoimmune thyroiditis and estrogen dominance, bind thyroid hormones to thyroid-binding proteins in the blood, making them unavailable for use by the cells. This is the reason that physicians should consider the patient's symptoms and signs as the primary basis for determining the diagnosis and subsequent treatment.

NATURAL DESICCATED THYROID HORMONE

As we saw in the Prelude, hypothyroidism (initially called myxedema) was recognized as a clinical disease by the physicians of the Clinical Society of London in 1888. In 1891 English physician Dr. George Murray injected the ground-up thyroid glands of sheep into a woman patient in her fifties, whom he had diagnosed with severe myxedema. The woman made a dramatic recovery. Eventually, she was given dried (desiccated) thyroid tissue and ultimately lived until 1921.

Over time, desiccated porcine thyroid glands (dried pig thyroid glands), were found to be the most prevalent and economical source of thyroid for treatment. As we've seen, natural desiccated thyroid has been used by physicians for well over 100 years safely, effectively, and economically. While Armour Thyroid has been the most commonly used desiccated thyroid hormone preparation, there are several other desiccated thyroid preparations, Westhroid and Nature-Throid, to name just two. Desiccated thyroid USP may also be prepared by a compounding pharmacy at the request of a physician who wants to vary the strength of the prescription or make sure that it contains no allergic additives, or both.

WHAT IT CONTAINS

Desiccated pork thyroid contains the prohormone, T4, the active hormone, T3, as well as T1 and T2, which are precursor thyroid hormones that affect the utilization of thyroid hormones within the cells.

WHICH FORM OF THYROID HORMONE REPLACEMENT IS BEST?

Synthroid (levothyroxine sodium) is the number-one prescribed treatment for hypothyroidism. In 2002 it was the fourth most-prescribed drug in the United States overall. But a drug's popularity is no guarantee of its efficacy.

I had been trained to use synthetic thyroid drugs myself, but when I spoke with Dr. Mabray at the 1992 Pan American Allergy Society conference, I asked him which product he used. Dr. Mabray told me that he treated hypothyroidism with Armour Thyroid, a natural prescription thyroid supplement that he felt was much more effective than the synthetic thyroid products. While I had great respect for Dr. Mabray, I thought it wise to seek a second opinion. For that, I turned to Dr. Dor Brown, the patriarch and cofounder of the Pan American Allergy Society.

Dr. Brown lived in Fredericksburg, Texas, and even though he was in his 80s, he had one of the largest allergy practices in the country. He was also one of the finest clinicians I have ever known. Although he was board certified in both ear, nose, and throat surgery and in ophthalmology, his practice was multifaceted. Patients traveled from all over the country seeking his medical expertise for a host of medical conditions. As I mentioned in Chapter 4, Dr. Brown felt Armour Thyroid was superior to synthetic thyroid replacement drugs—"Because it works!"

Our clinical experience in treating more than 25,000 patients with hypothyroidism over the past 20 years has convinced me that Dr. Brown was absolutely right. Because thyroid and allergic disorders often go hand in hand, I have had the opportunity to evaluate many patients for allergic disorders who were already being treated for hypothyroidism with synthetic thyroid. Most of these patients have had significant symptoms of low metabolic function, even while taking synthetic thyroid. Once these patients were converted to natural desiccated thyroid and given the appropriate dosage, their symptoms of hypothyroidism resolved.

ACTIVE TREATMENT

As noted in Chapter 4, many people languish on synthetic thyroid products because they contain only a synthetic version of T4, the inactive form of thyroid hormone. Taking T4 without T3 is like replacing only seven of the eight spark plugs in your car's engine. Your body's "engine" will run, but it will never function as well as it should.

In contrast, desiccated thyroid USP contains both of the thyroid hormone molecules that the body produces, T3 and T4, along with nutrients from the thyroid gland. Though many physicians mistakenly believe that Armour Thyroid, which is a manufactured desiccated thyroid product, is of inferior quality or variable potency, this FDA-approved product is formulated according to the exacting standards of the United States Pharmacopoeia (USP). To ensure that the product is consistently potent from batch to batch and tablet to tablet, analytical tests are performed on the raw material and the actual tablets.

T4 + T3 = IMPROVED MOOD AND COGNITION

Given the choice, most patients with hypothyroidism would prefer to take a thyroid hormone product that includes both T4 and T3. This isn't just my observation; it's the conclusion of a landmark study published in the *New England Journal of Medicine*.[85]

In this ten-week study, patients with hypothyroidism were randomized into two groups. One group received isolated T4 for the first five weeks and a combination of T3 and T4 for the last five weeks. In the second group, the sequence was reversed. All of the capsules looked alike, so the patients and their physicians were unaware of which treatment they were receiving during each five-week period. On the last day of each five-week period, patients were administered standardized psychological tests to assess their levels of depression, anxiety, anger, and other traits, as well as cognitive tests of memory, attention, learning, and other functions.

On six of 17 measures of mood and cognition, the combination of T4 and T3 proved superior to isolated T4. In particular, when patients received both thyroid hormones, their symptoms of fatigue, depression, and anger were significantly improved and they performed better on tests of attention, mental flexibility, and learning.

In addition to performing better on standardized tests, patients rated their own mood and physical symptoms as significantly improved on the combination product in comparison to isolated T4. When asked which treatment they preferred, the majority preferred the combination product, stating that they had more energy, could concentrate more easily, and simply felt better.

When patients received both T3 and T4 thyroid hormones, their symptoms of fatigue, depression, and anger were significantly improved, and they performed better on tests of attention, mental flexibility, and learning.

SYNTHETIC THYROID DRUGS:
A TARNISHED HISTORY

Effectiveness is an important criterion in choosing a thyroid replacement product. But equally important is the safety of the product. Here again, natural thyroid has proven superior. Natural desiccated thyroid extracts have been in use for more than a century and were approved by the FDA in 1939, a year after the passage of the Food, Drug, and Cosmetic (FDC) Act.

Despite the fact that T3 is the active thyroid hormone within our cells and that it is four (4) times more active than T4, drug companies began to synthetically produce thyroxine, T4, products because they could be inexpensively manufactured. Thyroxine was eventually patented under brands names such as Synthroid, Levo-throid, and Levoxyl, which are now the accepted treatment for hypo-thyroidism in the United States. Synthroid entered the market in 1955, more than 50 years after desiccated thyroid had been in use. The other synthetic thyroid hormones entered shortly thereafter. Huge marketing campaigns were initiated in order to promote these synthetic thyroid preparations. None of them had FDA approval because of the mistaken assumption that these products were not new drugs and that their manufacturers were not required to prove their safety or effectiveness.

INCREASED SCRUTINY

However, in 1997, the FDA ruled that oral levothyroxine sodium products were indeed "new drugs" and that manufacturers who wanted to continue marketing these products must submit a new drug application (NDA) for approval. This decision was based on a long history of potency and stability problems with these drugs. In fact, between the years 1991 and 1997, there were ten recalls of synthetic thyroid drugs, involving more than 100 million tablets. These recalls were initiated because the synthetic thyroid drugs had a lower potency than they claimed, or they had lost their potency before their expiration dates.[86]

Despite this tarnished history, most doctors continue to prescribe Synthroid and other brands of synthetic thyroid hormone and remain unaware of the benefits of desiccated thyroid USP, such as Armour Thyroid.

AGGRESSIVE MARKETING

If synthetic thyroid hormone costs twice as much and is less effective, why do conventional physicians continue to prescribe it? It seems that it must be due to the huge marketing campaigns of the pharmaceutical companies that hold patents on these drugs. On May 27, 2012, Abbott Laboratories, the manufacturer of Synthroid, received the American Association of Clinical Endocrinologists (AACE) Outstanding Corporate Partner Award at the AACE 21st Annual Scientific and Clinical Congress in Philadelphia. It is the AACE and its members that have been the most vociferous opponents of desiccated thyroid hormone. Now you understand why. If someone's action, or that of an organization, seems contrary to common sense, you need to look for the money trail.

Because naturally occurring substances, including desiccated thyroid hormone, cannot be patented, these products have a lower profit margin, and the companies that make them do not have millions of dollars at their disposal for marketing. It is a case of David versus Goliath, and in this case, it is Goliath, the pharmaceutical industry known as Big Pharma, that wins. As a result of pharmaceutical marketing, the patient is pushed aside and left to deal with her or his hypothyroid symptoms with more expensive, less effective synthetic thyroid drugs.

A TYPICAL REGIMEN

At our center we begin our patients on a very low dose of desiccated thyroid USP, usually half a grain (30 mg), and increase the dose incrementally over a period of weeks and even months while simultaneously monitoring the patient's level of improvement in symptoms. We also measure the amount of free thyroxine in the blood and the TSH to ensure they stay within a range that we consider safe. Because the ranges of thyroid blood tests are so broad, we can safely increase the dose of thyroid when indicated in order to enable the patient to reach her or his optimal level of thyroid. This process continues until the patient's symptoms are resolved.

VIEW ON THE GROUND

Our clinical experience indicates that many patients receive little or no relief of their hypothyroid symptoms when they take synthetic thyroid. We have evaluated thousands of patients who have presented to us with clinical symptoms of hypothyroidism while they were taking synthetic thyroid preparations.

There may be some individuals who have improvement on synthetic thyroid, but we do not see them at our center. We attract patients who have hypothyroid symptoms that have not resolved or in some cases worsened on synthetic thyroid therapy. This may give us a skewed view in the overall effectiveness of synthetic thyroid, but our clinical experience proves to us that many individuals do not benefit from synthetic thyroid medications.

MEDICAL OPPOSITION

By searching the Internet for hypothyroidism, you can find scores of websites and blogs where individuals are complaining about the ineffectiveness of synthetic thyroid and praising the benefits of desiccated thyroid USP. One of the best websites is www.thyroid. about.com, which is managed by Mary Shomon. She had struggled with undiagnosed hypothyroid symptoms for years. Eventually, she was able to find a physician who treated her with desiccated thyroid supplementation and her life dramatically changed. She has dedicated herself for over a decade to distributing information to hypothyroid individuals about the choices that exist for treatment with desiccated thyroid, which many doctors don't know about or simply discount.

Unfortunately, when doctors hear from their patients these complaints of hypothyroidism or of the ineffectiveness of synthetic thyroid medications, they usually turn a deaf ear and tell the patient that the blood work indicates that their hypothyroidism has been effectively treated. These physicians will often tell them that they are getting older and just have to learn to live with it. If patients complain too much, doctors will inform them that the problem is all in their head and that they are depressed, and they prescribe an antidepressant.

Why is it that most doctors will not listen to their patients' complaints when they tell their doctors that their synthetic thyroid treatment is not working? Why won't these physicians consider the possibility that their treatment might be ineffective and give their patients a clinical trial of desiccated thyroid USP?

Having healthy thyroid function is not always as simple as supplementing with thyroid hormone. There are a several factors that can affect the way that thyroid hormone is processed and utilized in the body. An imbalance of thyroid hormone rarely travels alone. There are additional pieces to the thyroid puzzle.

THE IMPORTANCE OF THE THYROID-ADRENAL CONNECTION

When considering treatment, it's important to bear in mind major points about the adrenal glands' influence on thyroid health that we covered in Chapter 4:

- The adrenal glands are like shock absorbers for stress. They cannot run on overload, and chronic stress, overstimulation, or an intense trauma can exhaust them.
- In addition to cortisol, the adrenals produce androgens such as DHEA that stimulate or control the development and maintenance of masculine characteristics. The adrenals also make aldosterone, which maintains blood pressure and balances the body's salt and potassium levels.
- Numerous hormones in your body direct what is known as your body's hormonal cascade. If one hormone fails, the rest of the cascade does not act properly. Cortisol, DHEA, and aldosterone are part of the hormonal cascade and work synergistically with the thyroid gland.
- Adrenal fatigue often occurs in conjunction with hypothyroidism and many of their symptoms overlap. Because thyroid and adrenal hormones work in concert, adrenal insufficiency can exacerbate hypothyroid symptoms. Adding supplemental thyroid hormone may

result in initial improvement in energy and a reduction in other symptoms. However, the adrenal glands may become even more exhausted, and this shuts down energy production altogether.

- The solution is not more thyroid hormone, but adrenal support with small doses of cortisol instead. In my experience, as well as that of Dr. Jefferies, bioidentical cortisol in small dosages improves vitality, raises body temperature, and increases resistance to infection. Cortisol also helps the body utilize thyroid hormone. Natural cortisol is especially helpful for patients with autoimmune thyroiditis.

- Like other autoimmune conditions, autoimmune thyroiditis can develop when the adrenal glands are stressed, especially following pregnancy or at menopause. As documented in Dr. Jefferies' book, natural cortisol actually reduces levels of thyroid antibodies, enhancing the effectiveness of thyroid hormone.

- Adrenal fatigue can also be part of the underlying cause of chronic fatigue syndrome and fibromyalgia.

BRINGING ALLERGIES INTO THE PICTURE

Chronic allergies are often a characteristic of hypothyroidism and adrenal fatigue. An allergy is an abnormal reaction by the immune system to normally occurring substances in our environment. Patients with allergies often experience the following:

- frequent headaches
- frequent colds or infections
- fatigue

- nasal symptoms such as sneezing, drainage, dripping, or constant itching
- eye symptoms such as itching, swelling, watering, or dark circles under the eyes
- recurrent and chronic sinus infections
- recurring cough or bronchitis
- asthma
- recurrent ear infections
- eczema, skin rashes, itching, and hives
- recurring yeast infections
- indigestion, bloating, constipation, diarrhea

If your symptoms occur seasonally, you may suffer from allergies. If you have a family history of allergies, it may be that you also have a family history of hypothyroidism. Allergy treatment desensitizes you to the common airborne allergies to which you react, such as weed, tree and grass pollens, dust mites, mold spores, and animal danders. Rather than merely masking the symptoms with antihistamines and decongestants, allergy desensitization therapy stimulates your immune system to develop antibodies that block the allergens to which you react.

DESENSITIZING AGAINST ALLERGENS

Allergens may be identified through skin testing or through a blood test. A custom formulation of allergy drops is prepared so that you can begin desensitizing yourself to your allergies. The treatment for allergy desensitization is sublingual. This means that you are able to take your allergy drops under your tongue instead of by injection. No more allergy shots!

LINK TO HYPOTHYROIDISM

Because of a weakened immune system, people with hypothyroidism are at a much greater risk for allergies and subsequent infections. Our approach normalizes the immune system that produces the allergic reactions. We optimize your thyroid and adrenal function while desensitizing your immune system to the common airborne allergens.

Many women without a history of allergies began experiencing allergies shortly after the birth of a child or during midlife. By listening to my patients, I discovered the relationship between hormone imbalance and the triggering of allergies. This commonly occurs during the transitional hormone stages of a woman's life, especially after childbirth. In order to treat the allergic disorder, the underlying hormonal problems must be addressed.

DEALING WITH FOOD ALLERGIES

Food allergies are also common among hypothyroid patients. To identify the offending foods, implement a food elimination/rotation diet to manage your allergies. You start with a one-month low allergenic diet, eating the following foods unless you have a reaction:

- chicken
- turkey
- beef
- pork
- fish
- lamb
- fresh vegetables
- beans
- rice

- potatoes
- salads with cold-pressed, virgin olive oil

Follow this diet for one month, and then add to your diet one new food at a time, in its purest form, every two days. Monitor for any symptoms that may occur. Sublingual drops may be used to neutralize allergy reactions. If symptoms do not appear, the food can be rotated into your diet every four or five days.

SEX HORMONES

Along with a decline in thyroid and adrenal hormones as we age, there is also a decline in our sex hormones. Most women believe that menopause is an isolated event, but actually it is preceded by up to 15 years of declining female hormones, particularly progesterone, which is associated with abnormal menstrual periods and breakthrough bleeding. As we've seen, because your estrogen, progesterone, and cortisol work in concert with thyroid hormone, an imbalance in your sex and adrenal hormones can affect your thyroid function, as well as the utilization of thyroid hormone by your cells.

As we have discussed, estrogen dominance leads to the production of TBG by the liver, which prevents thyroid hormones from being adequately assimilated into your cells where they can actually do their work of enabling the cells to produce energy. To balance estrogen dominance, bioidentical progesterone is needed.

Men aren't off the hook on this one. They suffer a decline in testosterone known as andropause. The hormonal change in men is gradual. It's the kind of thing where a man looks back on his life over the past few years and realizes that he has lost something. Maybe his drive and initiative just aren't what they used to be or his endurance and stamina have taken a hit. Men tend to gain only one thing in andropause: an inner tube around their middle. We simply replenish the hormones that are declining or missing altogether. It sounds too simple to fix what seems like a complex problem, but as I wrote earlier, more often than not, medicine isn't rocket science; it's common sense.

PRESCRIBING PROGESTERONE

Each woman is different, with her very own hormonal fingerprint, so the dosage varies accordingly. Premenopausal women take bioidentical progesterone on days 15 through 28 of their menstrual cycle. Postmenopausal women take progesterone every day. The reason for the difference in dosage is because as women age, their progesterone levels fall at a more dramatic rate than estrogen. The more mature you are in age, the greater the imbalance between your progesterone and estrogen levels.

YEAST OVERGROWTH

You have learned that candida albicans is a yeast or fungus that is normally present on the skin and in the mouth, throat, intestines, and in women it is also found in the vagina. The healthy bacteria in your intestines are killed by antibiotics, so yeast flourishes and grows out of control.

In addition to taking antibiotics, if you have ever eaten antibiotic-injected meat or dairy products, taken birth control pills, or steroids, you are susceptible to yeast overgrowth. Chlorine, fluoride, and nonsteroidal anti-inflammatory drugs (NSAIDS), such as aspirin and ibuprofen, all kill the healthy bacteria in your intestinal tract and when added to a diet loaded with sugar, we see the overgrowth of candida, fungi, mycoplasma, and anaerobic bacteria in our intestines.

This creates a condition of yeast overgrowth, called candidiasis, and it can affect virtually any organ in the body, causing a myriad of negative health symptoms including those that affect your thyroid. These organisms release neurotoxic chemicals into the bloodstream that damage the hypothalamus and alter thyroid production. Candida also increases autoimmune thyroiditis by disrupting the immune system and causing "friendly fire" against other organs in your body.

RESPONDING TO YEAST

In order to ensure that this is not negatively affecting the health of your thyroid gland and digestive tract, it is imperative that you remove excess yeast from your gastrointestinal system.

Our approach to ridding the body of yeast is a lot like pulling weeds in a garden. The first step is to kill the yeast with an antifungal drug called Nystatin. Nystatin has been in use for more than 50 years and is a safe, effective agent for eradicating yeast in the colon. It is not absorbed systemically, and it does not affect the beneficial bacteria that normally inhabit the colon. Fluconazole is a pharmaceutical drug that is also used to kill yeast in the colon lining.

The second step is to prevent yeast from regaining a foothold in your body. Otherwise, while you may win the battle, you will ultimately lose the war. We recommend a yeast-free, grain-free diet that eliminates dietary sources of yeast and other fungi, vinegar, and fermented products, and sugar and carbohydrate-rich foods that provide nourishment to yeast. Our cookbook, *The Hotze Optimal Eating Program*, outlines for our patients the guidelines of the diet as well as delicious recipes following the program.

The third step in ridding your body of yeast overgrowth is to replenish the good bacteria in your body. We must repopulate what years of antibiotic use have destroyed. We recommend taking probiotics, such as Lactobacillus acidophilus, to build up your good bacteria.

We encourage our guests at the Hotze Health & Wellness Center to participate in a two- to three-month, yeast-free eating program to ensure success. This not only eliminates sugar in the diet, decreasing the amount of inflammation in the body, but it also removes the source for possible toxins inhibiting your thyroid gland function.

VITAMINS AND MINERALS

Did you know that you can boost your thyroid function by adding a few vitamins and minerals to your supplement regimen? A vitamin and mineral foundation is critical to your overall health. Here are some of the elements it should include:

Quality multivitamin: The first step is to find a quality multivitamin that is free of allergens, harmful fillers, or sugars and that contains a full B complex without added iron. The B vitamins especially improve cellular oxygenation and energy and are needed for proper digestion, immune function, red blood cell formation, and thyroid function.

Vitamin D: Many hypothyroid patients have low levels of vitamin D. A deficiency in vitamin D increases your risk for major diseases such as cancer, heart disease, and osteoporosis. Have your physician check your 25-hydroxy vitamin D level and consider optimizing your vitamin D level.

Fish oil: Americans get way too many omega-6 fatty acids in their diet and not enough omega-3 fatty acids. Fish oil is a great source of omega-3 fatty acids, which are necessary for proper functioning of the thyroid gland.

Iodine: Hypothyroidism caused by iodine deficiency is characterized by a goiter, or enlarged thyroid gland. Although this no longer commonly occurs due to the use of iodized salt, most Americans still have low levels of iodine in their system, which adversely affects thyroid health. The thyroid hormone requires iodine. Supplemental iodine may stimulate thyroid hormone production.

Fluoride, chloride, and bromide are halogens that are common in our food and our water. These atoms are in the same family as iodine and inhibit iodine uptake. This is another reason for supplementing with iodine.

Selenium: Selenium is an antioxidant that helps convert T4, the inactive thyroid hormone, to T3, the active hormone, by cleansing the cells of harmful toxins that get in the way of proper conversion.

L-Tyrosine: Low blood levels of the amino acid L-Tyrosine are associated with hypothyroidism. L-Tyrosine is the amino acid that provides the backbone of thyroid hormone. It is important to make sure that your body has plenty of this amino acid on board.

SUMMARY

1. Factors that distinguish the Hotze Health & Wellness Center approach include listening carefully to guests, conducting a thorough clinical evaluation, regarding guests as partners in the journey to better health, always asking questions, treating guests with the utmost hospitality, building a community, and providing opportunities for continuing education and support.

2. Thyroid tests are not to be relied upon.

3. Our clinical experience has taught us that natural desiccated thyroid provides superior treatment over synthetic thyroid. A

thorough treatment regimen for hypothyroidism takes into consideration the thyroid-adrenal connection, allergies, sex hormones, yeast overgrowth, and nutritional supplementation.

4. For more information, please visit www.hotzehwc.com/TreatmentProgram.

chapter

ELEVEN

BEYOND TREATMENT: LIFELONG WELLNESS

One of the ways that I have chosen to spread the news about the wellness revolution in which we are fully engaged is to spend time with the ladies and gentlemen who have chosen to seek care and treatment at the Hotze Health & Wellness Center. These guests, many of whom are raving fans, have been active in their communities in telling their friends, family members, and acquaintances about the impact that thyroid treatment and other parts of our treatment program have had on their health and lives. As I mentioned in the last chapter, they are our ambassadors. Many of them have dramatically restored their health, which has transformed their lives and improved their worlds, naturally. Others have experienced significant improvement and are progressing along the pathway to health and wellness. Still others have experienced remarkable recoveries only to backslide, so to speak, into unhealthy habits and need to recommit themselves to following a lifetime change in their health habits. This leads me to make the following point.

Your body has been fearfully and wonderfully created by God. He has given your body amazing restorative power required to heal itself and flourish. As we mature, we experience ever-changing circumstances both within our bodies and in our lives that affect our health. As you initiate your treatment regimen, your body's requirements will invariably change over time. This will require adjustments to be made with your thyroid, bioidentical hormones, and your nutritional support. This requires that you listen to your body and communicate with your physician and his or her staff so that the appropriate adjustments can be made.

FINE-TUNING TREATMENT

It is only by listening to our patients that we are able to successfully manage their thyroid supplementation program over the long term. In some cases, we hear from individuals that they were doing great with our treatment until suddenly something changed. In cases like these, there are questions that our physicians ask to determine whether to lower or increase the thyroid dose or the dose of other bioidentical hormones:

1. How much thyroid was being taken at the time the symptoms appeared?
2. Were any supplements, medications, or hormones recently added, subtracted, increased, or decreased?
3. What dose of thyroid medication worked, and for how long, to resolve the previous symptoms?
4. Were any life events involved that increased stress levels, such as marriage, divorce, pregnancy, and so on?
5. Are any new pharmaceutical drugs being used?

Oftentimes what I have found is that the answers to these questions will provide insight for the best solution to the problem. Because each individual is completely different, the solution will always be unique for that individual. Here are some signs and symptoms that might have their genesis in the amount of thyroid hormone being used:

HEART ARRHYTHMIA AND/OR RACING HEART

When guests who have been doing well on their thyroid protocol tell me they have begun to experience an increase in heart rate or heart palpitations, this may be an indication that the dose of thyroid medication needs to be lowered. Often by simply stopping the thyroid preparation until the symptoms resolve and then returning to the previous dose of thyroid medication when these symptoms are absent corrects the problem.

DIFFICULTY LOSING WEIGHT

An individual who has achieved optimal health and wellness generally does not have an issue maintaining an ideal body weight. Therefore, when someone suddenly starts to experience difficulty in this area, altering the dosage of thyroid may be required. In our practice, we see this most often in our guests who have been on an effective hormone supplementation and eating program for a number of years. As we age, our bodies sometimes require increasing amounts of the hormones to maintain an ideal state. It is obvious that someone who is 55 may require more thyroid hormone than someone who is 35. Therefore, we ask a lot of questions to ensure that the guest has maintained a nutritious and balanced eating program. If so, we allow the individual to increase his or her thyroid dosage in small increments until the metabolism increases sufficiently to allow maintenance of a healthy and active lifestyle.

IN HER OWN WORDS: AMY'S STORY

Even as a child, I probably started having problems with my thyroid at a very young age. I think at the age of 11 or 12, I actually asked my mom for Jenny Craig at Christmas because my weight was an issue for me, although I was active in at least three or four different sports throughout the year. I was a very active child, but weight was always a concern of mine. I continued to play sports through college and still had the weight issue. The older I got, the worse it seemed to be.

Early Diagnosis but No Resolution

I was prescribed thyroid medicine at the age of 16, once it was confirmed that I had a thyroid problem. I was on Synthroid at a very low dose. It took a lot of convincing for them to even put me on that—regular doctors—because they felt that even though my number was on the low end of the 1–10 scale, it was still active. I was on thyroid for many, many years and it was going nowhere. The older I got, the worse my health became.

In 2003 I started seeing specialists because doctors couldn't figure out what was going on with me. I started taking medications for prediabetes. My pancreas was working about 20 times the amount of a normal person. I was having problems with my liver. I was having problems, and my whole body was beginning to shut down. In total, I went to at least 11 specialists, the majority of them being in the Medical Center here in Houston. Nobody could figure out what was going on with me.

The reason I ended up coming to the Hotze Health & Wellness Center is because I had been seeing a specialist for two years. I had seen some improvements with this specialist, but she finally told me, "There are so many things going on with you. I can't figure them out. You are going to have to see someone else because I've done all I can for you."

Host of Difficulties

This doctor's recommendations had helped a little bit, but, for example, Metformin, one of the drugs she gave me, had ten possible side effects. I had every one of them.

Headaches, cramping, gas, diarrhea, upset stomach—I had these on a daily basis. It was not pretty. But with that, I started to feel a little bit better, compared to where I had been previously. When I say a little bit better—it was mild, because I was going down the drain. Sort of like, if this is living, this is not the way I want to live. I could no longer wake up on my own. I'd set four or five alarms around my bedroom, and they'd all have to go off for me to get out of bed. I'd get into the shower. I'd fall asleep in the shower. I'd get out of the shower, try to get ready for work, and I'd fall asleep again. I had the hardest time trying to get up and get going. On top of thyroid issues, I had adrenal failure. Complete adrenal failure. But I didn't find that out until Dr. Sheridan evaluated me.

None of my other doctors had run any tests on me. On top of being extremely tired, I had put on an extreme amount of weight. I was eating, literally, like a salad or two a day, and fruit. All healthy, but I was gaining five to six pounds a week. I had so much water retention that it was hard to move. I was sore all the time and achy. My body was storing everything. Dr. Sheridan later explained to me that the problems with my thyroid created a domino effect for me. So the problems with my metabolism led to additional problems with my adrenal function, which led to problems with my liver.

I didn't know where to turn because my doctor said she was at a loss as to who to refer me to. My life was a mess. I was trying to pass my second bar. I was trying to work, but I was miserable. I began feeling depressed, though I fought it every day. I was fighting to stay awake. It got to the point where I would have to take a nap during my lunch break, and then a nap right after work, because if I didn't, I couldn't make it home. It didn't matter if I got eight hours, 10 hours, 12 hours of sleep; I still could not function. My body was literally shutting down, and my life outside of work was nonexistent.

Receiving Care

By the time I finally came to see your doctors at the Hotze Health & Wellness Center, I was in a state of emergency. I had struggled with the decision to come in for a little while, but eventually I knew it was something I had to try.

When I saw Dr. Sheridan, he took a lot of time to listen to my previous history during his assessment. Because I had so many different issues, we agreed to try one thing at a time and slowly, gradually keep adding things to help. He switched me from Synthroid to Armour Thyroid right away. Within the first two weeks, I could see a major change for me. Two weeks! When I started seeing results, it was like the light at the end of the tunnel, and I was full-steam ahead to get there. Over the next few weeks, we would progressively add a little bit more thyroid medicine. Then he advised me to start taking cortisol, which we also added more of, a little at a time. I also eventually began taking progesterone because

I had developed polycystic ovary disease. Throughout it all, I ate yeast free because I was determined to get where I wanted to be. I had progressively put on weight since high school, and after about a year under Dr. Sheridan's care, I lost 70 pounds!

One of the things I most appreciate about the Hotze Center is that as my life changes and my symptoms change, we make adjustments. In that first year, I was in frequent contact with the nurses at the office to make small tweaks to what I was taking. I would describe what I was experiencing; they would listen to me, ask lots of questions. We would assess the dosages of the hormones or supplements, and make decisions together about what to change. It feels like I have a partner for life who will help me stay on this path of health.

Amy's story clarifies an essential part of working to obtain and maintain optimal health—namely, that communication with the medical team is crucial to be able to quickly solve issues that can arise from time to time. Fatigue, hair loss, difficulty losing weight, depressed moods, heart palpitations—these are some common symptoms that may reoccur at some point during the process of thyroid hormone supplementation. They often occur years after successfully starting treatment, though sometimes they can unexpectedly arise earlier. In each instance, tweaking the original dose that brought about symptom relief with the possible addition of certain nutrients generally solves the problem and restores hormonal balance, as it did and continues to do in Amy's case.

CONCLUSION

By now it should be abundantly clear that hypothyroidism is responsible for a myriad of serious conditions that can substantially decrease the quality of life and in many cases, shorten it.

It still stuns me, after all of these years, to have the sheer volume of patients who come to us with a wide range of health issues that have not been properly addressed by their physicians. Instead, they have been prescribed everything from statin drugs to antidepressants, drugs that have side effects and only mask symptoms.

Unfortunately, we are very often our guests' last resort. The good news is that when they do find us, we are able to help them.

The reason I wrote this book is so that you would have the information to empower you to make healthy, substantial changes in your life. Thyroid supplementation appropriately prescribed and monitored by a physician can be life changing.

At the Hotze Health & Wellness Center, our goal is to transform lives.

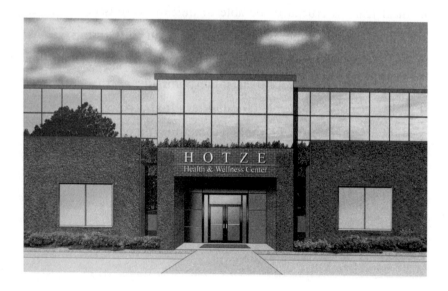

We know that when people get their health back, they also get their families back and their lives back. One day we will reach a tipping point at which the medical community will finally acknowledge that pharmaceutical drugs are not the best solution for improving your health. Until then, we will continue to advance the wellness revolution, educating and encouraging people, one by one.

YOUR OWN WAY FORWARD

The stories of the patients in this book are true. Although many of them suffered for years before finally being diagnosed, they have made dramatic improvements and are now finally able to live their lives in an exceptional fashion. You have your own story to tell, and my hope is that you will also be successful in restoring your health, transforming your life, and improving your world naturally.

Do you have hypothyroidism? There is a simple checklist in Appendix A that can help you to begin the discovery process.

My goal for you is that if we were to meet one year from now, you would be on a path of health and wellness and you would be able to dream and live again. There is power in the spoken word, and in the written word. Make a contract with yourself to change your life for the better. Fill out the contract below, sign it, date it, and post it where you can see it every day.

A CONTRACT WITH YOURSELF

I, _____, will make the necessary changes so that I can get my health and my life back. I will listen to my body and will find a physician who is supportive of natural desiccated thyroid hormone supplementation and understands that hypothyroidism is diagnosed through clinical symptoms, not a lab test. I owe it to myself, my family, and my friends to be healthy and well. My life is important.

Signature: _____

Date: _____

DEBBIE'S STORY

As a final thought, I leave you with the words of another guest, who chose to express her experiences in verse.

My story, like yours,
Has been pretty bad.
I could go on about
Troubles I have had,
The nights without sleep,
The days with no peace,
The doctors I've sought,
And the remedies bought.
All of this to no avail;
I felt like I was in a jail
Of fear and pain and feeling bad
And never knowing what I had.
The "experts" said, "your tests are fine.
All of this is in your mind.
Antidepressants—that's the key."
WELL NOT ANYMORE—NOT FOR ME!
Thank you God
For getting me through,
And showing me folks
Who know what to do.

Drs. Hotze, Sheridan, and their crew
Said, "You're not alone, there's hope for you."
So, I followed advice and did what they said
And just like I thought—IT'S NOT IN MY HEAD.
This is amazing; this is great.
Life shouldn't end at twenty-eight.
My son has his mom back; my husband, his wife,
And I'm ready again to start living my life.
If this sounds like you
And you're lost and upset,
Give Hotze a call—
They'll help YOU, I bet!

SUMMARY

1. Your body has God-given restorative powers.

2. Listening is a key not only to determining a successful course of action for our guests, but to making appropriate adjustments that continually fine-tune treatment.

3. You need to take positive steps to protect your own health, and I encourage you to make a written commitment to do so.

4. For more information, please visit www.hotzehwc.com/ArtOfListening and www.hotzehwc.com/RealSuccessStories.

APPENDIX A

Do you have
Low Thyroid Function?
(hypothyroidism)

Read each question carefully and check the box if it applies to you.
*When you finish, give yourself **one point** for every check to total your score.*

☐ Do you have fatigue?

☐ Do you have elevated cholesterol?

☐ Do you have difficulty losing weight?

☐ Do you have cold hands and feet?

☐ Are you sensitive to the cold?

☐ Do you have difficulty thinking?

☐ Do you find it hard to concentrate?

☐ Do you experience brain fog?

☐ Do you have poor short term memory?

☐ Do you have depressed moods?

☐ Are you experiencing hair loss?

☐ Do you have less than one bowel movement a day?

☐ Do you have dry skin?

☐ Does your skin itch in the winter?

☐ Do you have fluid retention?

☐ Do you have recurrent headaches?

☐ Do you sleep restlessly?

☐ Are you tired when you awaken?

☐ Do you have afternoon fatigue?

☐ Do you experience tingling or numbness in your hands or feet?

☐ Do you have decreased sweating?

☐ Have you had problems with infertility or miscarriages?

☐ Do you have recurrent infections?

☐ Do your muscles ache?

☐ Do you have joint pain?

☐ Do you have thinning of your eyebrows or eyelashes?

☐ Is your tongue enlarged with teeth indentations?

☐ Is your skin pasty, puffy or pale?

☐ Do you have decreased body hair?

☐ Is your voice hoarse?

☐ Do you have a slow pulse?

☐ Do you have low blood pressure?

☐ Does your body temperature run below the normal 98.6°?

☐ Do you have sleep apnea?

Total Score

☐ < 9 — It is not likely that you have low thyroid function.
9-28 — Low thyroid function is a possibility.
> 28 — Low thyroid function is very likely.

H O T Z E
HEALTH & WELLNESS CENTER

www.hotzehwc.com

ABOUT THE AUTHOR

STEVEN F. HOTZE, MD, received his medical degree from the University of Texas Medical School in 1976. In the 1980s he began to explore alternative ways to treat his father's heart disease, searching for real solutions beyond the drugs and surgery that had already failed his father. The safe, effective, nondrug treatments that he discovered enabled his father to live eight more productive years and revolutionized Dr. Hotze's approach to medicine.

In 1989 Dr. Hotze founded the Hotze Health & Wellness Center in Houston, Texas, in order to offer a revolutionary approach to optimal health, centered around listening to the patient and providing natural therapies, such as thyroid supplementation, bioidentical hormones, allergy immunotherapy, nutritional supplementation, and a balanced, healthful eating program. Over the years, tens of thousands of patients have come to the Hotze Health & Wellness Center to improve their health and enjoy a better quality of life.

In 2005 Dr. Hotze published *Hormones, Health, and Happiness*, and since then, more than 85,000 copies have been sold and distributed.

Dr. Hotze is a fellow member of the American Academy of Otolaryngic Allergy, past president of the Pan American Allergy Society, and founder and president of the American Academy of Biologically Identical Hormone Therapy (AABIHT). Dr. Hotze has trained numerous physicians in his proven, effective methods for enabling women in midlife to regain their health, increase their energy, and reclaim their lives.

Dr. Hotze and the other physicians at the Hotze Health & Wellness Center host a radio program, *Health and Wellness Solutions*, broadcast in Houston on AM 700 KSEV, Monday through Thursday from 12 noon to 1 p.m. central time, and on the web at www. ksevradio.com.

ENDNOTES

[1] Centers for Medicare and Medicaid Services. *National Health Care Expenditures Data*. Office of the Actuary, National Health Statistics Group, January 2012.

[2] Martin, A. B., D. Lassman, B. Washington, and A. Catlin, and the National Health Expenditure Accounts Team. "Growth in US Health Spending Remained Slow in 2010: Health Share of Gross Domestic Product Was Unchanged from 2009," *Health Affairs*, vol. 31, no. 1 (January 2012): 208–219.

[3] P. B. Ginsburg. "High and Rising Health Care Costs: Demystifying U.S. Health Care Spending." Princeton, NJ: Robert Wood Johnson Foundation, October 2008.

[4] Barnes, Broda O. *Hypothyroidism: The Unsuspected Illness*. New York: Harper & Row Publishers, 1976.

[5] Lowe, J. C. "Stability, Effectiveness, and Safety of Desiccated Thyroid vs. Levothyroxine: A Rebuttal to the British Thyroid Association," *Thyroid Science*, vol. 4, no. 3 (2009): C1–12.

[6] Cohen, R. A. and P. F. Adams. "Use of the Internet for Health Information: United States, 2009," Centers for Disease Control and Prevention, August 7, 2012, http://www.cdc.gov/nchs/data/databriefs/db66.htm.

[7] Rho, M. H., H. P. Hong, Y. M. Park, M. J. Kwon, S. J. Jung, Y. W. Kim, and T. Kang. "Diagnostic Value of Antithyroid Peroxidase Antibody for Incidental Autoimmune Thyroiditis Based on Histopathologic Results," *Endocrine*, May 2012 (Epub. ahead of print).

[8] Rambhade, S., A. Charkarborty, A. Shrivastava, U. K. Patil, and A. Rambhade. "A Survey on Polypharmacy and Use of Inappropriate Medications," *Toxicol. Int.*, vol. 19, no. 1 (2012): 68–73.

[9] National Center for Complementary and Alternative Medicine. "The Use of Complementary and Alternative Medicine in the United States," December 2008, accessed August 7, 2012, http://nccam.nih.gov/news/camstats/2007/camsurvey_fs1.htm.

[10] Lazarou, J., Pomeranz, B.H., Corey, P.N., "Incidence of Adverse Drug Reactions in Hospitalized Patients: A Meta-Analysis of Prospective Studies," *J Am Med Assoc*, Vol. 279, No. 15: 1200-05.

[11] Andersen, S., K. M. Pedersen, N. H. Bruun, and P. Laurberg. "Narrow Individual Variations in Serum T4 and T3 in Normal Subjects: A Clue to the Understanding of Subclinical Thyroid Disease," *J. Clin. Endocrinol .Metab.*, vol. 87, no. 3 (2002): 1068–72.

[12] Hollowell, J. G., N. W. Staehling, W. D. Flanders, W. H. Hannon, E. W. Gunter, and C. A. Spencer. "Serum TSH, T4, and Thyroid Antibodies in the United States Population (1988–1994): National Health and Nutrition Examination Survey (NHANESIII)," *J. Clin. Endocrinol. Metab.*, vol. 87, no. 2 (2002): 489–99.

[13] Centers for Disease Control and Prevention. "Congenital Hypothyroidism," accessed June 25, 2012, http://www.cdc.gov/ncbddd/pediatricgenetics/key_findings.html.

[14] American Association of Clinical Endocrinologists. "Blue Paisley Ribbon Introduced as the New Symbol for Thyroid Awareness," accessed October 31, 2012, http://media.aace.com/press-release/blue-paisley-ribbon-introduced-new-symbol-thyroid-awareness.

[15] Centers for Disease Control and Prevention. "National Diabetes Fact Sheet, 2007," accessed August 7, 2012, http://www.cdc.gov/diabetes/pubs/pdf/ndfs_2007.pdf.

[16] CBS News. "The Cost of Dying," December 3, 2010, accessed August 7, 2012, http://www.cbsnews.com/2100-18560_162-5711689.html.

[17] Gharib, H., R. M. Tuttle, H. J. Baskin, L. H. Fish, P. A. Singer, and M. T. McDermott. "Consensus Statement: Subclinical Thyroid Dysfunction: A Joint Statement on Management from the American Association of Clinical Endocrinologists, the American Thyroid Association, and the Endocrine Society," *J. Clin. Endocrinol. Metab.*, vol. 90, no. 1 (2005): 581–85.

[18] Arem, Ridha. *The Thyroid Solution: A Revolutionary Mind-Body Program for Regaining Your Emotional and Physical Health.* New York: Ballantine Books, an imprint of The Random House Publishing Group, a division of Random House, Inc., 2007.

[19] Glenmullen, Joseph. *The Antidepressant Solution.* New York: Free Press, Division of Simon & Schuster, 2005.

[20] Kharrazian, Datis. *Why Do I Still Have Thyroid Symptoms?* Garden City: Morgan James, 2010.

[21] Schumacher, M., R. Hussain, N. Gago, J. P. Oudinet, C. Mattern, and A. M. Ghoumari. "Progesterone Synthesis in the Nervous System: Implications for Myelination and Myelin Repair," *Front. Neurosci.*, vol. 6, no. 10 (2012) (Epub. ahead of print).

[22] Cowan, L. D., L. Gordis, J. A. Tonascia, and G. S. Jones. "Breast Cancer in Women with a History of Progesterone Deficiency," *Am. J. Epidemiol.*, vol. 114, no. 2 (1981): 209–17.

[23] Dandona, P. and M. T. Rosenberg. "A Practical Guide to Male Hypogonadism in the Primary Care Setting," *Int. J. Clin. Pract.*, vol. 64, no. 6 (2010): 682–96.

[24] Hajjar, R. R., F. E. Kaiser, and J. E. Morley. "Outcomes of Long-Term Testosterone Replacement in Older Hypogonadal Males: A Retrospective Analysis," *J. Clin. Endocrinol. Metab.*, vol. 82, no. 11 (1997): 3793–96.

[25] Jefferies, W. M. *Safe Uses of Cortisol*. Springfield, IL: Charles C. Thomas, 2004.

[26] Kaltsas, G., A. Vgontzas, and G. Chrousos. "Fatigue, Endocrinopathies, and Metabolic Disorders," *PMR,* vol. 2, no. 5 (2010): 393–98.

[27] Mizokami, T., A. Wu Li, S. El-Kaissi, and J. R. Wall. "Stress and Thyroid Autoimmunity," *Thyroid*, vol. 14, no. 12 (2004): 1047–55.

[28] Brownstein, David. *Iodine, Why You Need It, Why You Can't Live Without It*. West Bloomfield, MI: Medical Alternatives Press, 2009.

[29] de Benoist, B., F. McLean, M. Andersson, and L. Robers. "Iodine Deficiency in 2007: Global Progress since 2003," *Food and Nutrition Bulletin*, vol. 29, no. 3 (2008): 195–202.

[30] WHO Nutrition. "The WHO Global Database on Iodine Deficiency," accessed June 21, 2012, http://www.who.int/vmnis/en/.

[31] Starr, Mark. *Hypothyroidism, Type 2, The Epidemic*. Columbia: Mark Starr Trust, 2005.

[32] Coleman, R. and R. J. Hay. "Chronic Mucocutaneous Candidosis Associated with Hypothyroidism: A Distinct Syndrome?" *Br. J. Dermatol.*, vol. 136, no. 1 (1997): 24–29.

[33] Roger, V. L , Go, A.S., Lloyd-Jones, D.M., Benjamin, E.J., Berry, J.D., Borden, W.B., Bravata, D.M., Dai, S., Ford, E.S., Fox, C.S., Fullerton, H.J., Gillespie, C., Hailpern, S.M., Heit, J.A., Howard, V.J., Kissela, B.M., Kittner, S.J., Lackland, D.T., Lichtman, J.H., Lisabeth, L.D., Makuc, D.M., Marcus, G.M., Marelli, A., Matchar, D.B., Moy, C.S., Mozaffarian, D., Mussolino, M.E., Nichol, G., Paynter, N.P., Soliman, E.Z., Sorlie, P.D., Sotoodehnia, N., Turan, T.N., Virani, S.S., Wong, N.D., Woo, D., Turner, M.B., on behalf of the American Heart Association Statistics Committee and Stroke

Statistics Subcommittee. "Heart Disease and Stroke Statistics—2012 Update: A Report from the American Heart Association," *Circulation*, vol. 125 (2012): e2–e220.

34 Parle, J. V., P. Maisonneuve, M. C. Sheppard, P. Boyle, and J. A. Franklyn. "Prediction of All-Cause and Cardiovascular Mortality in Elderly People from One Low Serum Thyrotropin Result: A 10-Year Cohort Study," *Lancet*, vol. 358, no. 9285 (2001): 861–65.

35 Linder, F. E and R. D. Grove. *Vital Statistics Rates in the United States 1900–1940.* Washington, DC: United States Government Printing Office, 1947.

36 Anderson, R. N. and H. M. Rosenberg. *Report of the Second Workshop on Age Adjustment.* National Center for Health Statistics, Vital Health Statistics Series 4, no. 30. Washington, DC: United States Government Printing Office, 1998.

37 Heberden, William. "Description of Angina Pectoris," accessed June 12, 2012, http://rwjms1.umdnj.edu/shindler/heberden.html.

38 Mackenzie, James. *Diseases of the Heart.* London: Henry Frowde, Hodder & Stoughton, 1908.

39 Barnes, B. O., M. Ratzenhofer, and R. Gisi. "The Role of Natural Consequences in the Changing Death Patterns," *J. Am. Geriatr. Soc.,* vol. 22, no. 4 (1974): 176–79.

40 Pauling, L. and M. Rath. "Hypothesis: Lipoprotein(A) Is a Surrogate for Ascorbate," *Proc. Natl. Acad. Sci.,* vol. 87 (1990): 6204–7.

41 Rath, Matthias. *Why Animals Don't Get Heart Attacks but People Do.* Santa Clara: MR Publishing, 2000.

42 Gelb, Douglas J. "Hypothyroidism: Historical Note and Nomenclature," accessed July 16, 2012, http://www.medmerits.com/index.php/article/hypothyroidism/P1.

43 Stabouli, S., S. Papakatsika, and V. Kotsis. "Hypothyroidism and Hypertension," *Expert Review of Cardiovascular Therapy,* vol. 8, no.11 (2010): 1559–65.

44 Dawber, T. R., F. E. Moore, and G. V. Mann. "Coronary Heart Disease in the Framingham Study," *Am. J. Public Health Nations Health,* vol. 47, no. 4, pt. 2 (1957): 4–24.

45 Wren, J. C. "Symptomatic Atherosclerosis: Prevention or Modification by Treatment with Desiccated Thyroid," *J. Am. Geriatr. Soc.,* vol. 19, no. 1 (1971): 7–22.

46 Asvold, B. O., L. I. Vatten, T. I. Nilsen, and T. Bjoro. "The Association between TSH within the Reference Range and Serum Lipid Concentrations in a Popu-

lation-Based Study: The HUNT Study," *Eur. J. Endocrinol.*, vol. 156, no. 2 (2007): 181–86.

[47] Rodondi, N., Newman, A.B., Vigginghoff, E., de Rekeneire, N., Satterfield, S., Harris, T.B., Bauer, D.C. "Subclinical Hypothyroidism and the Risk of Heart Failure, Other Cardiovascular Events, and Death," *Arch. Int. Med.*, vol. 165 (2005): 2460–66.

[48] Hurxthal, L. M. "Blood Cholesterol and Thyroid Disease—III: Myxedema And Hypercholesterolemia," *Arch. Intern. Med.*, vol. 53, no. 5 (1934): 762–81.

[49] Barnes, B. O. "Prophylaxis of Ischaemic Heart-Disease by Thyroid Therapy," *Lancet*, vol. 274, no. 7095 (1959): 149–52.

[50] Kountz, W. "Thyroid Function and Its Possible Role in Vascular Degeneration," American Lecture Series, no. 108. Springfield, IL: C. C.Thomas, 1951.

[51] Virchow, R. *Die Cellularpathologie in ihrer Begründung auf physiologische und pathologische (Cellular Pathology as Based upon Physiological and Pathological History)*. Berlin: August Hirschwald, 1858.

[52] Konstantinov, I. E., N. Mejevoi, and N. M. Anchkov. "Nikolai N. Anichkov and His Theory of Atherosclerosis," *Tex. Heart Inst. J.*, vol. 33 (2006): 417–23.

[53] *USA Today.* "Cholesterol Guidelines Become a Morality Play," accessed July 24, 2012, http://www.usatoday.com/news/health/2004-10-16-panel-conflict-of-interest_x.htm.

[54] Behar, S., Graff, E., Reicher-Reiss, H., Boyko, V., Benderly, M., Shotan, A., Brunner, D. "Low Total Cholesterol Is Associated with High Total Mortality in Patients with Coronary Artery Disease," *Eur. Heart J.*, vol. 18 (1997): 52–59.

[55] Ellison, Shane. *The Hidden Truth About Cholesterol-Lowering Drugs*. s.l.: Health Myths Exposed, 2006.

[56] American Heart Association. "About Cholesterol," accessed August 20, 2012, http://www.heart.org/HEARTORG/Conditions/Cholesterol/AboutCholesterol/About-Cholesterol_UCM_001220_Article.jsp.

[57] *Wikipedia.* "Cholesterol," accessed August 20, 2012, http://en.wikipedia.org/wiki/Cholesterol.

[58] Saul, S. "Pfizer to End Lipitor Ads by Jarvik," *The New York Times,* February 26, 2008, accessed July 24, 2012, http://www.nytimes.com/2008/02/26/business/26pfizer.html?_r=1.

[59] Graveline, Duane. *Lipitor, Thief of Memory.* s.l.: self-published, 2006.

[60] Rosenbaum, D., J. Dallongeville, P. Sabouret, and E. Bruckert. "Discontinuation of Statin Therapy Due to Muscular Side Effects: A Survey in Real Life," *Nutr. Metab. Cardiovasc. Dis.*, June 28 , 2012 (Epub. ahead of print).

[61] Fischer, C., Wolfe, S.M., Sasich, L., and Lurie, P. "Petition to Require a Box Warning on All Statins," accessed July 24, 2012, http://www.citizen.org/hrg1588.

[62] Food and Drug Admdinistration (FDA). "Adverse Events Reporting System (AERS) Patient Outcomes by Year," accessed July 24, 2012, http://www.fda.gov/Drugs/GuidanceComplianceRegulatoryInformation/Surveillance/AdverseDrugEffects/ucm070461.htm.

[63] Hak, A. E., H. A. Pols, T. J. Visser, H. A. Drexhage, A. Hofman, and J. C. Witteman. "Subclinical Hypothyroidism Is an Independent Risk Factor for Atherosclerosis and Myocardial Infarction in Elderly Women: The Rotterdam Study," *Ann. Intern. Med.*, vol. 132, no. 4 (2000): 270–78.

[64] Centers for Disease Control and Prevention. "Overweight and Obesity: Adult Obesity Facts," accessed July 24, 2012, http://www.cdc.gov/obesity/data/adult.html.

[65] Food Pyramid. "MyPyramid," accessed July 24, 2012, http://www.foodpyramid.com/.

[66] O'Connor, K. A., R. J. Ferrell, E. Brindle, J. Shofer et al. "Total and Unopposed Estrogen Exposure across Stages of the Transition to Menopause," *Cancer Epidemiol. Biomarkers Prev.*, vol. 18, no. 3 (2009): 828–36.

[67] Centers for Medicare & Medicaid Services. "National Health Expenditure Data," accessed July 24, 2012, http://www.cms.hhs.gov/NationalHealthExpendData/25_NHE_Fact_Sheet.asp.

[68] Schumm-Draeger, P. M. "Diabetes Mellitus and Frequently Associated Endocrine Diseases," *MMW Fortschr. Med.*, vol. 148, no. 37 (2006): 47.

[69] Witek, P. R., J. Witek, and E. Pankowska. "Type 1 Diabetes-Associated Autoimmune Diseases: Screening, Diagnostic Principles and Management" (article in Polish), *Med. Wieku Rozwoj.*, vol. 16, no. 1 (2012): 23–34.

[70] AERS (Adverse Events Reporting System) Patient Outcomes by Year. *www.fda.gov.* [Online] [Cited: July 24, 2012 .] http://www.fda.gov/Drugs/GuidanceComplianceRegulatoryInformation/Surveillance/AdverseDrugEffects/ucm070461.htm.

[71] Food and Drug Administration (FDA). "Text of the Prescription Drug Marketing Act of 1987," accessed July 25, 2012, http://www.fda.gov/RegulatoryInformation/Legislation/FederalFoodDrugandCosmeticActFDCAct/Significan-

tAmendmentstotheFDCAct/PrescriptionDrugMarketingActof1987/ucm201702. htm.

[72] Bulik, B. S. "Ad Spending: 15 Years of DTC." In *Pharmaceutical Marketing* (white paper), 2011, October 17. accessed July 25, 2012, http://gaia.adage.com/ images/bin/pdf/WPpharmmarketing_revise.pdf.

[73] Sax, J. K. "Financial Conflicts of Interest in Science," *Ann. Health Law,* vol. 21, no. 2 (2012): 291–327.

[74] Drugs.com. "Tamoxifen Side Effects," 2012, accessed July 25, 2012, http:// www.drugs.com/sfx/tamoxifen-side-effects.htm.

[75] Maugh, T. H. "Banned Report on Vioxx Published," *Los Angeles Times,* January 25, 2005, accessed July 25, 2012, http://articles.latimes.com/2005/jan/25/ science/sci-vioxx25.

[76] Angell, M. *The Truth about the Drug Companies: How They Deceive Us and What to Do About It.* New York: Random House, 2004.

[77] Centers for Disease Control and Prevention. "Fibromyalgia 2011," 2011, accessed July 25, 2012, http://www.cdc.gov/arthritis/basics/fibromyalgia.htm

[78] Wolfe, F., Clauw, D.J., Fitcharles, M.A., Goldenberg, D.L., Katz, R.S., Mease, P., Russell, I.J., Winfield, J.B., Yunus, M.B. "Preliminary Diagnostic Criteria for Fribro-myalgia and Measurement of Symptom Severity," *Arthritis Care & Research,* vol. 5 (2010): 600–10.

[79] Rubenstein, S. "Pfizer and Lilly Plow Marketing Money into Fibromyalgia," *The Wall Street Journal,* February 9, 2009, accessed July 25, 2012, http://blogs.wsj.com/health/2009/02/09/ pfizer-and-lilly-plow-marketing-money-into-fibromyalgia/.

[80] Sahay, R. K. and V. S. Nagesh. "Hypothyroidism in Pregnancy," *Indian J. Endocri-nol. Metab.,* vol. 16, no. 3 (2012): 364–70.

[81] Stagnaro-Green, A. "Maternal Thyroid Disease and Preterm Delivery," *J. Clin. Endocrinol. Metab.,* vol. 94, no. 1 (2009): 21–25.

[82] Chen, I. "Pregnancy and the Thyroid," *The New York Times,* March 13, 2009, accessed July 25, 2012, http://www.nytimes.com/ref/health/healthguide/esn-hypothyroidism-expert.html?pagewanted=all.

[83] Negro, R., G. Formoso, T. Mangieri, A. Pezzarossa, D. Dazzi, and H. Hassan. "Levothyroxine Treatment in Euthyroid Pregnant Women with Autoimmune Thyroid Dissease: Effects on Obstetrical Complications," *J. Clin. Endocrinol. Metab.,* vol. 91, no. 7 (2006): 2587–91.

[84] Shomon, M. J. "David Derry, M.D., Ph.D., Re: TSH Tests," accessed July 25, 2012, http://thyroid.about.com/od/thyroiddrugstreatments/l/blderryb.htm.

[85] Bunevicius, R., G. Kazanavicius, R. Zalinkevicius, and A. J. Prange Jr. "Effects of Thyroxine as Compared with Thyroxine Plus Triiodothyronine in Patients with Hypothyroidism," *New Engl. J. Med.*, vol. 340, no. 6 (1999): 424–29.

[86] "Prescription Drug Products; Levothyroxine Sodium." *Federal Register*, vol.62, no. 157 (14 August 1997) accessed February 15, 2013, http://www.gpo.gov/fdsys/pkg/FR-1997-08-14/pdf/97-21575.pdf.

INDEX

A

AACE (American Association of Clinical Endocrinologists), 239

Abilify, 174

ACE inhibitors, 172

ADA (American Diabetes Association), 165

Addiction and antidepressants, 183

Adenosine triphosphate (ATP), 61

Adrenal fatigue, 48, 110–114, 219–220, 242–243

Adrenal hormones

    aging and, 83, 109, 246

    cholesterol, 143

    infertility, 214

    miscarriage, 214

    online information, 230

    statin drugs, 146

    thyroid-adrenal connection, 114, 242–243

Adrenaline, 110–111

Adverse reactions to prescription drugs, 41, 57

Advertising and polypharmacy, 172–174

Aging

adrenal hormones and, 83, 109, 246

arthritis and, 83

cancer and, 83

desiccated thyroid, 109

heart disease, 83, 109

hormones and, 83–85, 109

hypertension, 83, 109

obesity, 83

sex hormones and, 83–84

Agriculture Department, U.S., 162

Allergies, 48, 243–246. See also Food allergies

Alternative medicine, 40

Alzheimer's disease, 24, 83, 109

Ambien, 174

American Association of Clinical Endocrinologists (AACE), 239

American College of Rheumatology, 200–202

American Diabetes Association (ADA), 165

Andropause, 108–109, 246–247

Angell, Marcia, 187

Angina pectoris, 131–132, 137

Anitschkow, N., 140–141

Antibiotics. See also Probiotics

Y

Z